PRIMARY NURSING

Person-Centered Care Delivery System Design

SUSAN WESSEL & MARIE MANTHEY

CREATIVE

HEALTH CARE

MANAGEMENT

Library of Congress Cataloging-in-Publication Data
Wessel, Susan, 1952- , author.
Primary nursing : person-centered care delivery system design / Susan Wessel, Marie
Manthey.
    p. ; cm.
Preceded by: Practice of primary nursing / Marie Manthey. 2nd ed. c2002.
Includes bibliographical references and index.
ISBN 978-1-886624-15-3 (pbk. : alk. paper)
I. Manthey, Marie, author. II. Manthey, Marie. Practice of primary nursing. Preceded by
(work): III. Creative HealthCare Management (Minneapolis, Minn.), issuing body. IV. Title.

[DNLM: 1. Primary Nursing. WY 100.1]
RT102
610.73--dc23

                            2015022903

Softcover ISBN 13: 978-1-886624-15-3
ebook ISBN 13: 978-1-886624-96-2

Printed and bound in the United States of America.

19 18 17 16 15   6 5 4 3 2

Second Printing: October 2015

Cover and interior design by James Monroe Design, LLC.

For permission and ordering information, write to:
Creative Health Care Management, Inc.
5610 Rowland Road, Suite 100
Minneapolis, MN 55343

www.chcm.com
800.728.7766 / 952.854.9015

CREATIVE
HEALTH CARE
MANAGEMENT

Dedication

This book is dedicated to Florence Marie Fisher, a nurse who cared for me when I was hospitalized at the age of five with scarlet fever, in St. Joseph's Hospital, Chicago. Although I never saw her again, her personalized and very humane care of me became a model that I have followed throughout my life and professional career.

This dedication is also made to all those nurses who recognize the profound influence this special kind of nursing practice can have on the lives of their patients and who, by practicing it themselves, preserve the proud tradition and invaluable legacy of all of the nurses like Ms. Fisher, which is ultimately the highest tribute of all.

MARIE MANTHEY

This book is also dedicated to the first organization I joined as a new graduate nurse, Rush Presbyterian–St. Luke's Medical Center in Chicago. I was hired in a unit just beginning Primary Nursing. Nursing at Rush proved to be an exquisite introduction to professional practice. I learned what it meant to accept ownership for leading the care of patients as a Primary Nurse, and I felt the fulfillment of having that special bond with patients. The legacy of Luther Christman, Nurse Executive extraordinaire, and his successor, Sue Hegyvary, proved to be the perfect environment to begin a career. Rush was far ahead of its time with clinical ladders, shared governance, and Primary Nursing. I will always consider myself a "Rush nurse."

SUSAN WESSEL

Contents

Part III: Best Practices and Sustainment Strategies

Acknowledgments

First and foremost, we'd like to thank the seven Primary Nurses who allowed us to interview them about their work and to use their responses in this book. We know that it is their words that will inspire readers more than anything else, but the value of their contribution to the two of us, as we assembled this book, cannot be overstated. It is fortunate that they were so eloquent because the avalanche of validation of the value of this work that came out of those interviews left us speechless. These Primary Nurses, identified as exemplars by their managers, are Jane Czekajewski, BSN, RN, CNOR; Kathleen Fowler, BSN, RN; Kelly Lehmkuhl, BSN, RN, OCN; Kirsten Roblee, BSN, RN, OCN; and Dena Uscio, BBA, RN, OCN, of The Ohio State University Comprehensive Cancer Center—Arthur G. James Cancer Hospital and Richard J. Solove Research Institute (OSUCCC—James); and Heidi Nolen, BSN, RN; and Nicole Vance, BSN, RN, of UC Davis Medical Center in Sacramento, California.

Our heartfelt gratitude goes to developmental editor Rebecca Smith for amplifying and beautifying the content of this book. She approached her work on this book with one audacious aim: that everyone who reads it would become an evangelist of Primary Nursing.

Numerous other people had a hand in ensuring that this book would fulfill its dual purpose of helping readers understand the essential role Primary Nursing plays in any culture that presumes to be relationship-based or patient-centered and in instructing readers in the hands-on implementation of Primary Nursing. We'd like to thank Chris Bjork for project management; Jay Monroe for designing the cover and interior of the book; Marty Lewis-Hunstiger, BSN, RN, MA, and Mary Koloroutis, MSN, RN, for editing assistance; and Fred Dahl, Cathy Perrizo, and Kary Gillenwaters for proofreading assistance.

We'd also like to thank Mary Koloroutis and Michael Trout for every word of *See Me as a Person: Creating Therapeutic Relationships with Patients and Their Families* and for their generosity in allowing us to use their content in Chapter 7 of this book. We'd also like to thank Creative Health Care Management consultants Mary Griffin Strom and Janet Weaver for their contributions of the stories featured in Chapter 7 and the Epilogue, respectively.

Finally, we wish to acknowledge all of the talented people who have made significant contributions to professionalizing nursing in hospitals in the 1970s. Only a few people, however, will be mentioned here specifically. Beginning in the early 1970s, June Werner of Evanston Hospital in Evanston, Illinois, and Joyce Clifford of Beth Israel Deaconess Medical Center in Boston implemented Primary Nursing with such integrity that the level of professional practice achieved during their tenure stands as an eternal flame, forever reminding us of the importance of leadership. More recently, Carol Robinson at UC Davis Medical Center in Sacramento, Georgia Persky at New York–Presbyterian Hospital/Columbia University Medical Center in New York City, and Susan Brown and Jamie Ezekielian at OSUCCC—James in Columbus have demonstrated sustained and comprehensive implementation of Primary Nursing with stellar outcomes.

Part I
Why Primary Nursing?

I've been kind of shocked at the patient feedback in the audits. I remember assessing whether one gentleman knew who his Primary Nurse was, and he named her right away. I asked him what kind of difference it has made and if there was anything he wanted me to know about the kind of care she was giving him. He got choked up and couldn't even talk. You can't ask for anything better. He was so moved by the things we do here. He was so appreciative of everything.

—Kelly Lehmkuhl, bsn, rn, ocn
Primary Nurse at OSUCCC—James

Primary Nursing is Your Most Direct Route to a Better Health Care Experience

As we approached the writing of *Primary Nursing: Person-Centered Care Delivery System Design*, we were struck by the vast difference between what it's like to write about a care delivery system only a decade or so after its invention and writing about it after it has been practiced not merely adequately, but beautifully, for well over four decades all over the world. It is no longer necessary to spend ink on dispelling the myths and misknowings associated with Primary Nursing. While its merits as a care delivery system may still be a mystery to many of those who have not yet experienced it firsthand, it has proven to be nothing short of a miracle to the hundreds of thousands who have.

Primary Nursing was born directly out of the dissatisfaction that one group of nurses was experiencing in their professional roles. They began to see, too clearly for comfort, that functional and team nursing systems were designed to accommodate caregivers and those supervising caregivers, not patients and their families. In what amounted to a collective flash of insight, a small group of like-minded nurses realized not only that patients and families weren't getting what they needed most—the unshakable knowledge that one smart, capable person has accepted responsibility for their care—but that they were working in an environment where the systems and processes that shaped activities on the unit were working against their ability to show up as professionals and accept responsibility for anything beyond compliance with rules and regulations. We will never know exactly how many nurses said, "This is not right," before the small off-campus gathering took place that gave birth to Primary Nursing. The world of nursing changed subtly but inexorably that day, when a group of nurses on Unit 32 at the University of Minnesota Hospital recommended to Marie Manthey that they try a new way of providing care. Marie said yes, taking a risk. She was wise enough to have experts study the new delivery system and measure its impact right from the start. Primary Nursing was born, and it was quickly shown neither to cost more nor to require any changes in staffing or skill mix.

We have all come a long way since then. The obstacles those first nurses had to overcome to design and practice Primary Nursing are beyond what anyone implementing Primary Nursing will ever have to deal with again.

Still, when we talk with nurses practicing Primary Nursing today, their excitement at the prospect of redesigning how care happens on their units is no less immediate than the excitement experienced by those who pioneered it. Even on units where Primary Nursing finds itself in the doldrums because of new initiatives or other factors threatening to derail it, nurses who understand Primary Nursing go to great lengths to save it. We have seen repeatedly that nurses who have practiced Primary Nursing are never again completely content to practice within a less person-focused system of care, and the incontrovertible truth is that all other systems of care delivery are less person-focused than Primary Nursing.

In preparing to write the much anticipated follow-up to Marie Manthey's seminal work, *The Practice of Primary Nursing*, we interviewed seven nurses selected by their managers as exemplary Primary Nurses. In these interviews, we were struck by something that happened in every encounter: As nurses spoke about the logistical realities of Primary Nursing, they dutifully told us about patient assignment algorithms, color-coded teams, and other scheduling practices that have worked well on their units. Later in the interviews, when we asked them about the impact of Primary Nursing on their patients and families, they exhaled deeply, smiled (audibly), and told us story after story about the difference it makes to their patients. When we asked them about the impact it has on nurses, we got a similar response. Their gratitude for the privilege of getting to know their patients as people and to really deeply understand each patient's condition was evident in every interview. They are more respected by their team members—particularly their physician team members—because they are highly knowledgeable about their patients. They are experiencing the satisfaction that is known only by those who are willing to enter into the privilege of accepting responsibility for leading the care of another person. We know that if you haven't experienced it firsthand, it's hard to imagine it. That is the challenge in writing this book.

Perhaps you should hear about Primary Nursing from those who are practicing it every day:

On the Impact of Primary Nursing on Unit Culture

Kirsten Roblee, bsn, rn, ocn

In a high-stress situation you know the patient so well that you rattle off their history without having to dig through their chart. We are very knowledgeable because we are so entrenched in our patients' treatment and care. In critical situations, being able to see the team at their best helps build mutual respect on the unit.

On the Impact of Primary Nursing on Patient Safety

Kathleen Fowler, bsn, rn

I have a patient who refers to me as "My Katie." I've taken care of her almost sixteen times straight, so I know her very very well. If she came in and had just a subtle change—say she had nausea—it might not be a red flag to anybody else, but it's going to be a red flag to me because it's something new for her. Primary Nursing allows you to give safer care because you might catch something early on. I think that's one of the highlights of Primary Nursing; it sets the patient up to get better care.

Dena Uscio, bba, rn, ocn

We had a medication issue with a patient where they may have gotten too big a dose. The Primary Nurse knew the patient's home dose and was able to adjust it so that we wouldn't spend all this money doing all this testing (and delay correcting the problem) when the Primary Nurse already knew what the cause was.

Nicole Vance, bsn, rn

We've had kids being taken care of by float nurses who didn't know anything about them, and the kid radically deteriorated. It was only when someone who knew the child walked by the room that somebody said, "Wait a minute, that's not how that child is supposed to look." And a doc might say, "Well, hold on, that still could be his baseline ..." Maybe he's a very developmentally delayed child, so it can be hard to know. One of the benefits of Primary Nursing is that you have a guaranteed person to say, "No! This is not his baseline; where he's at now is dangerous, and if we don't nip it in the bud, we have about two hours before we'll be sending him to the ICU."

On Primary Nursing as a Means to Create a Safe Haven for Patients and Families

Heidi Nolen, bsn, rn

It really takes almost a whole shift to get families to even want to talk to you and trust you, and if we give them different nurses every day, they never really get the feeling of a trusting relationship or safety in the hospital. Once the relationship is established and they understand my role and the commitment that goes with it, the parents feel confident that it's okay to leave their child with me and go and nurture their other relationships and take care of themselves. Even if it's just to go get some coffee or have breakfast, it's the security in knowing that I am giving their child the right medications—and that, yes, I do sincerely love their child, and they know that if they walk away for a second everything will be okay.

On Nurse–Physician Relationships, Professionalism, and Advocacy

Nicole Vance, bsn, rn

Nothing will turn a specialist's head like a Primary Nurse respectfully disagreeing about something based on six years of experience with the patient and family. The docs want to hear that. The continuity, the time with the family—that's time they don't get. They get 15 minutes at a time with the patient, and they know that someone who has had hours and hours and hours with them will have a perspective that is pure gold. We've had Primary Nurses change the tide of a patient's entire hospital course because of one fact they found out from a grandparent in the hallway.

Kelly Lehmkuhl, bsn, rn, ocn

The physicians see what strong advocates we are and how much we care. They see the great relationships we develop with our patients and how that makes us go the extra mile. I think the Primary Nursing role in general has really increased our autonomy as nurses, our self-confidence, our decision making. Physicians see how we are in our role, and it inspires confidence. It didn't happen overnight, but once we developed the consistency of the team and physicians could see our competence and commitment, over time they developed greater trust in us.

Kirsten Roblee, bsn, rn, ocn

Our nurse–physician relationships were always great. The attending would tell the interns, "You need to listen to the nurses because they're going to save your butts." Now that they've experienced our role in Primary Nursing, the level of respect the physicians show nurses has increased. They include us in more lengthy, in-depth conversations. There is more collaboration. Instead of talking with us about patient care on a surface level, physicians are talking about the specific strains found in blood cultures and educating us on what to expect with each strain. We have more influence now because we know the patient's history, in-depth knowledge of lab and test results, etc. Growth on the relational side is obvious but is now apparent on the technical side; we have a bigger part of taking care of the patients.

On Primary Nursing Being Easier Than Other Systems of Nursing

Dena Uscio, bba, rn, ocn

In the beginning, our little tagline to "sell" Primary Nursing to our staff was, "Primary Nursing isn't about doing more; it's about being more." It worked because it's true. We're not adding tasks. There's not another step. It's about being more involved. It's easier for the charge nurse to make

> "Primary Nursing isn't about doing more; it's about being more."

5

assignments because it takes out the whole question of where to start, and it lays out a whole framework on how to make the assignment. For the Primary Nurse, it's easier because you know these patients. You know their preferences, you can anticipate their needs, and you can help physicians; it can really make your day easier.

Heidi Nolen, bsn, rn

There may be a time when I have four primary patients on the unit, and I wonder whether I'll be capable of caring for all of them because of the acuity. A lot of times, for me personally, even with the acuity, I'd be more open to taking care of those patients I've had as primaries before because I already know them and that's half the battle. Sometimes half the challenge of being busy is just not knowing the family dynamics or their preferences, so I would still rather care for them even if the acuity was higher because I've already established the relationship.

On the Impact of Primary Nursing on Patients and Families

Kirsten Roblee, bsn, rn, ocn

It's comforting for the patients to know that they have one nurse who is a consistent participant in their care. On our unit, the attending doctors change every two weeks and Nurse Practitioners change every two days, causing anxiety in many patients. The Primary Nurse is the most consistent person in their hospital stay, and they all verbalize that it's very comforting. They know who is on their side; they don't have to look through their caregivers' business cards at a time when that's the last thing they want to do. Our name is on the board; sometimes our picture is in the room; they know who we are.

Jane Czekajewski, bsn, rn, cnor

I think it's great that we can go up and see our patients after surgery. It kind of gives the OR Primary Nurse a connection because it's nice to be able to convey, "I took care of you for ten hours... but you didn't really know it." So again we're building the relationship, and people are really moved that the nurses are reinforcing that connection.

Kathleen Fowler, bsn, rn

We have a really good relationship, and a lot of times that's why our patients want to come in here by themselves. They're out in the community and people feel bad for them, and the patients almost end up taking care of the people who are in grief over their condition. But they can come in and I'm here, and for that period of time, they can have not one worry in the world. Sometimes they cry with me or other members of their team because they can't cry with their spouse. That's big. It's not like they would cry with every nurse; it's because we have a relationship. They cry with us because we're "family," but we're family they don't have to take care of.

Dena Uscio, bba, rn, ocn

I've had patients cry when I explain who I will be to them as their Primary Nurse. A lot of our patients are coming in with a new diagnosis. They've got a cough that won't go away and all of a sudden they're diagnosed with cancer. They're scared, they're vulnerable, and we are telling them, "I am here for you. You have support in here. You have someone you can ask questions of. You have someone who will help interpret all of this medical craziness that you don't understand." That act of saying, "I am your Primary Nurse," to the patient—I have had families cry. It's been a wonderful reaction.

Is that what nursing looks like in your organization?

As you begin to have conversations with colleagues at all levels about Primary Nursing, here is what you will discover: Those who have experienced it firsthand tend to be enthusiastic advocates of it, and those who have not experienced it firsthand can be pretty negative about it. "It's too hard," they will tell you, having never done it.

In 1980, Marie Manthey published the first edition of *The Practice of Primary Nursing*. One of the most satisfying aspects of her long career has been assisting strong, capable nurse leaders in their efforts to establish Primary Nursing on their units and in their organizations. Over that long tenure, she and her consultant colleagues have seen nurses at every level of licensure overcome seemingly insurmountable obstacles because they understood the value of the work they were doing to create and nurture an infrastructure that provided the time, space, and systems for relationships with patients and their families to flourish and team relationships to deepen into gratifying partnerships.

Primary Nursing: Person-Centered Care Delivery System Design, written more than 35 years later, is a new book for a new generation of nurses. The concepts are the same, the work is the same, and the same level of commitment and persistence are necessary, but the world has changed, and nurses have changed and are still changing.

We spend a lot of time with nurses of all ages. We know what they're thinking because we ask them about it. What we see in this current generation of nurses, as exemplified by the voices of the nurses you just heard, is a deepening of the commitment, which has always existed to some degree in nurses, to connect authentically with the patients and families in their care. There is often nothing in the experience of these nurses to suggest that there is *time* for authentic connection. It seems, however, that this generation of nurses intuitively knows that they will simply not survive in the profession if they don't figure out how to create and sustain meaningful relationships with their patients and families, as well as with each other. Nurses used to tolerate poor collegial relationships because they thought they had to. Nurses used to tolerate impersonal, task-based nursing practice because they didn't know there was a better way. Things are changing. Many nurses are hungry for a reconnection to the meaning and joy in their profession.

This book was written to address the changes we are seeing in health care, in nursing, and in nurses themselves. New information has been added to address the myriad advances that have been made in Primary Nursing due to its expansion into milieus such as ambulatory and surgical settings, as well as into interdisciplinary departments. Because brilliant, tenacious staff nurses all over the world have embarked on the work of designing and practicing Primary Nursing since the late 1960s, the body of knowledge has grown significantly.

Still, nursing is for the most part practiced within largely bureaucratic institutions, and these institutions, like most of the rest of the developed world, are operating under a "domination paradigm" (Eisler & Potter, 2014). If you work in the world of health care, you probably readily acknowledge that there are hierarchies within your organization. What you may not so readily acknowledge is that those hierarchies may also exist in your own mind. Because you were born into a domination paradigm, unless you've consciously worked to change this paradigm within yourself, it's very likely that you view the world through a domination paradigm lens without even realizing you're doing so.

In *Primary Nursing: Person-Centered Care Delivery System Design*, care has been taken to ensure that rather than a domination paradigm, it is a partnership paradigm that is reflected. A partnership paradigm doesn't mean a flat org chart; hierarchies still exist in a partnership paradigm. What's different is the *way of being* of the people involved. You know when you're being partnered with, and you know when you're being dominated. The much harder thing to notice, however, is when *you* are—sometimes ever so subtly (and perhaps even "for the greater good")—being the dominator.

As we look at Primary Nursing through the lens of the partnership paradigm, it comes alive in new ways. Primary Nursing is and has always been about creating healthy partnerships between nurses and other clinicians in order to best serve patients and their families. As we approach this work with all of the implications of partnership in the front of our minds, we are reminded of the adage, "How I do anything is how I do everything." Since the goal is for Primary Nurses to forge productive, empowered, inspired partnerships with patients and families, the system in which these partnerships are expected to exist must be created by a group of productive, empowered, inspired partners. The core of Primary Nursing is a therapeutic partnership with patients. If this is what the unit or organization desires, it must then actively support the creation of systems and processes that promote this relationship every step of the way.

Chapter 1

The Historic Ebb and Flow of Nurse Autonomy

Marie Manthey

Adapted from *The Practice of Primary Nursing* (1980, 2002, updated 2015).

Primary Nursing in acute care hospitals is a delivery system for nursing at the department level that facilitates person-centered professional nursing practice despite the bureaucratic nature of hospitals. The practice of any profession is based on an independent assessment of a person's needs, which determines the kind and amount of service to be rendered. Services in bureaucracies are usually delivered according to routine preestablished procedures without sensitivity to variations in needs. In bureaucracies, functions are grouped into service lines or departments and headed by leaders who usually retain decision-making authority.

Here's where Primary Nursing comes in: For professional nurses to thrive within a bureaucracy, the system used to deliver care must be designed to minimize the bureaucratic impact and maximize the empowerment, accountability, and authority of professional nurses.

Within a bureaucracy, many different delivery systems may coexist to accomplish the numerous functions of the various

> *For professional nurses to thrive within a bureaucracy, the system used to deliver care must be designed to minimize the bureaucratic impact and maximize the empowerment, accountability, and authority of professional nurses.*

departments. These systems will support either bureaucratic or professional values, depending largely on the design of the system and the philosophy of leadership in the organization. Before Primary Nursing was established at the University of Minnesota in 1968, the delivery systems used for hospital nursing reflected bureaucratic rather than professional values. Both functional nursing systems (in which one nurse passes all medications, another does all treatments, and several people give all baths) and team nursing systems were designed according to a mass-production model of service delivery; the least complex tasks are assigned to the least trained workers, the more complex to more skilled workers, and so on up a hierarchy of task complexity. In those systems, registered nurses were assigned two functions: (1) to administer the most complex tasks and (2) to coordinate and supervise the tasks done by the lesser prepared workers. Registered nurses in this system were not professional caregivers; rather, they were "checker-uppers of cheaper-doers." This sort of dynamic might make great sense in a factory setting in which temporary workers are asked to do unskilled work, but in the world of nursing where critical thinking and experience are extremely valuable, it is an unconscionable misapplication of talent. Also, nowhere in this formula is room made for the nurse to establish a therapeutic relationship with the patient.

Primary Nursing is a delivery system that creates the opportunity for nurses to develop a professional role in which their technical and relational skills are equally valued and supported. In short, a care delivery system will either actively support nurses in the full expression of their professional roles or contribute to the deprofessionalization of nursing.

There are four characteristics generally agreed on by sociologists as descriptive of the ways a profession can be differentiated from another endeavor or occupation. They are

1. An identifiable body of knowledge that can best be transmitted in a formal educational program.

2. Autonomy of decision making.

3. Peer review of practice.

4. Identification with a professional organization as the standard setter and arbiter of practice.

Clearly, nursing has an identifiable body of knowledge, peer review of practice, and identification with an appropriate professional organization. It is most often the extent to which the second characteristic—autonomy of decision making—is supported within an organization that determines whether the professionalism of nursing is being promoted or undermined. This support cannot just be lip service. Again, an organization's care delivery design will facilitate autonomous decision making by professional nurses, or it will contribute to the deprofessionalism of nursing.

Deprofessionalization continues to be a major problem, not only in nursing but within other professions as well. In the last four decades, macro political and economic changes have profoundly influenced society, health care, and nursing. The three most prominent drivers of change were financial, regulatory, and technological factors. Health care in the United States became a business rather than a social program. For-profit hospitals, multihospital systems developed through mergers and acquisitions, complex reimbursement schemes, and elaborate marketing campaigns became the visible signs of system changes in the 1980s and 1990s. In the early 21st century, economic recession and a major reform of the health care system drove us back to centralized decision making. Integrated health systems and Accountable Care Organizations have multiplied in an effort to bring the full continuum of care under one structure. Large numbers of uninsured people and intense competition among health care systems have driven revenues down, while health care costs overall continue to rise faster than the GNP as a whole. Reimbursement regulations drive clinical decisions and reduce the autonomy of physicians and other health professionals. Standardized care protocols and financial/government regulations erode professional autonomy in every allied health discipline. Thus, the deprofessionalization that nurses first experienced when their practice moved into hospitals is now being experienced by people in many professions within and outside of the health care system.

> *An organization's care delivery design will facilitate autonomous decision making by professional nurses, or it will contribute to the deprofessionalism of nursing.*

How the Pendulum Has Historically Swung Between Task-Based and Relationship-Based Nursing

The history of nursing from the 1870s to the 1930s marks the slow evolution of the nurse from practicing with the autonomy and whole-patient focus that characterize private duty nursing to practicing in salaried positions as employees of bureaucratic institutions.

The earliest period of nursing in the United States, from the 1870s until the Great Depression, was somewhat paradoxical in that task-based nursing was exclusively used in hospitals where nursing education took place and most of the care was delivered by student nurses. The majority of registered nurses in that era were employed as private duty nurses for individuals in private homes, a setting which is inherently relationship-focused. In the late 1930s, when large numbers of these nurses moved from private duty back to hospital-based nursing, they must have felt as though they had taken a full step backward professionally because they had all at one point literally graduated from the task-based practice they experienced as student nurses to the relationship-based practice of private duty nursing. In this era, the pendulum swing from relationship-based practice to a focus on tasks was driven by the migration of nursing back into a bureaucratic setting.

It is important to note that nurses did not come into these institutions by choice. Since it was the Great Depression that caused the displacement of these private duty nurses, many of them initially worked in hospitals for no wages, just room and board. Eventually they would be paid a stipend of just $5/month. Because they entered into these bureaucratic institutions in positions of utter powerlessness, they did what they were told to do and they did it the way they were told to do it, or they faced disciplinary action. The emphasis was on maintaining order.

That's what it's like in a domination paradigm. At that point in our history, it did not seem to occur to anyone to partner with or engage the collective wisdom of a group of women in the workforce, no matter how competent or experienced they were. Even women in positions of authority didn't dare to breech the unwritten rules of this rigidly hierarchical paradigm because to do so was to jeopardize their own positions of authority and, in fact, their livelihoods.

Most professional leaders believed that as soon as the Great Depression was over, these RNs would go back into private duty. Instead, of course, the

United States entered World War II, and the whole system of health care changed dramatically.

Changes in the health care system during and after WWII can be summarized as follows:

- The complexity of care increased exponentially due to technological advances.

- Hospitalization insurance was provided by employers to attract employees during the severe wartime labor shortage, and hospitalization rates increased.

- Large numbers of ancillary workers were trained during the war, and care delivery systems were designed to incorporate these lesser prepared caregivers into patient care.

These developments and many others resulted in the phenomenal growth of the health care system in complexity and size. Further fueling this growth, federal grants and low interest loans made available by the Hill-Burton Act of 1946 were available for hospital expansions and for the construction of new hospitals. At that time, there was a sense that there would never be enough hospital beds to meet the need. The unprecedented building boom put enormous pressure on human resources. An early fear that military nurses would return to American hospitals and flood the labor market, thus reducing salaries, was not borne out in reality. Instead the opposite occurred. The post–World War II era was heralded as a "return to normal," when women left their wartime employment, got married (or stayed married), stayed home, and had babies. This combination of a wave of young women leaving the field of nursing and the subsequent population explosion resulted in a dire nursing shortage.

Team nursing became the care delivery model of the era. In fact, in order for a school of nursing to be accredited by the National League of Nursing, it had to be affiliated with a hospital that was practicing team nursing. In team nursing, RNs continued to perform the unfortunate role of checker-uppers of cheaper-doers, and ultimate responsibility for each patient was transferred to a different RN every shift, none of whom had an incentive to learn about who the patients were or what they were experiencing. The shared responsibility in team nursing may sound both democratic and fair, but in nursing, shared responsibility essentially means that no one is responsible. The team leader assigned all tasks but was also accountable for making sure that everything was done on time. A team member who failed to perform a certain procedure when it was due could say to the team leader, "You forgot to remind me." This sharing of responsibility for performing care tasks meant that if something was not done, no one person was truly accountable.

> In nursing, shared responsibility essentially means that no one is responsible.

Team nursing is something that evolved because of changes in the settings in which nursing was practiced and in response to an influx of lesser prepared caregivers after the war. It provided a practical fix for the exact problems it addressed, and the nurses working within the system were too overworked and underempowered to spend much time assessing its pros and cons. It was a care delivery system designed to make things easier for nurses and the people who supervised nurses; it wasn't designed to address what patients and families wanted and needed.

I entered nursing school in 1953, so this is where the story of the pendulum swing between task-based practice and relationship-based practice becomes a firsthand account. Like nearly all of my peers, I spent from 1953 all the way through most of the 1960s as an obedient, eager-to-please, well behaved nurse. But there were rumblings in our culture during that time that were making their way into nursing, and while there were always people who pushed to keep things the way they were, there was eventually too much "power to the people" thinking in the culture to completely ignore the fact that we were far from empowered, even when it came to the things we knew better than those who were denying us the power to do them.

In my own life, from 1961 to 1968, I had an education going on in my house that was far better than anything I could have gotten in school. My then husband was a political science and philosophy major, and I typed his papers, read a fair number of his books, and took part in lots of discussions. I was introduced to a great variety of thinkers, and I became less blind in my obedience and much more open-minded. I attended community meetings, read radical authors, and went to protests, but always with one foot planted firmly in the system.

A real turning point came in 1966, when John Westerman became the director of University Hospitals and Clinics at the University of Minnesota. He was brought in to guide a big expansion project, and he and his associates taught me about decentralization and the fundamentals of how complex systems work. They opened a new way of thinking that became, for me, a new way of looking at just about everything.

When it became my job to develop ways to improve the practice of nursing at the direct care level in our institution, I looked at the issue through a systems lens as well as through the lenses of all of the authors I was reading at the time. At that time, author and social critic Paul Goodman talked about centralized and decentralized decision making. He pointed out that when the product being created requires a knowledge-based worker because of its unpredictability, you needed someone with the knowledge to handle that unpredictability, but when you're looking for a mechanized outcome, decision making can be centralized without ill effect. It was suddenly obvious to me that health care was and always will be characterized by the kind of unpredictability that makes decentralized decision making necessary. At about that same time, author Jay Hall made a big impression on me with the idea that people who design work systems typically organize for incompetence. We assume incompetence, build systems to accommodate it, and set them in motion; if instead we organized so as to expect people to be competent, we would foster competence. It's easy to see how all of this would prepare the soil for Primary Nursing and also provide all of us with the intellectual capital necessary to take what Primary Nursing was on day one and mold it into what would eventually become a sustainable care delivery system.

In 1966, when I was an assistant director doing special projects at the University of Minnesota Hospital, I read a journal article that, in my opinion, provided nurses with their first real invitation to create for themselves a more professional practice. It was called "Existentialism: A Philosophy of Commitment," written by Sister Madeleine Clemence and published in the *American Journal of Nursing* (1966). In this piece, Sister Madeleine, who was both a nurse and a philosopher, spoke of the difference between moving through life as a spectator and deciding instead to be *involved* with the people and situations with whom we come into contact. She wrote:

In existentialism, commitment means ... a willingness to live fully one's own life, to make that life meaningful through acceptance of,

rather than detachment from, all that it may hold of both joy and sor-
row. (Clemence, 1966)

Remember, this is a nurse talking. When she's talking about "acceptance of, rather than detachment from, all that life may hold," she's talking
about accepting and staying fully present to some things that may be very
hard to bear. As a nurse herself, she knew that the work of the nurse is
sacred, but it is sacred only for those who are really committing themselves
to being present with people in their suffering.

It was a radical call to action, particularly for nurses working within
systems in which they were expected to be obedient, dispassionate workers
as opposed to capable, authentic human beings with critical thinking abil-
ities. Here was Sister Madeleine challenging us to look at whether we were
simply "solving problems" as task-focused nurses or truly entering into the
mystery of what it means to be with people who are suffering, vulnerable,
and afraid. She quotes philosopher Gabriel Marcel: "A mystery is a reality
in which I find myself involved ... whereas a problem is [merely] in front of
me" (Clemence, 1966). This article appeared just as many of us were seeing
how infantilizing much of the bureaucracy we worked within really was.
Hospital leaders certainly weren't encouraging us to bring our authentic,
critically thinking selves to work, but we were beginning to figure out that
they couldn't actually stop us from doing so either.

Reaching the Boiling Point

In 1968, I was project director on Unit 32 at the University of Minnesota
Hospital. Like every reputable hospital in the United States, we were doing
team nursing, but the world was changing, and the nurses on Unit 32 were
changing with it. The unrest in the culture at large shook things loose, and
the empowerment we were finding in the women's liberation movement
was beginning to mobilize us in ways that nothing previously had.

I was appointed to co-direct a project designed to improve the delivery
of hospital departmental services to the nursing units. We conducted several studies to collect baseline data so that innovations could be evaluated
for their cost savings and effectiveness. For over a year, multiple projects
were conducted, and many of those piloted were quickly implemented
throughout the hospital.

A major goal for this project was to reduce the amount of time nurses spent in non-nursing activities to improve the quality of patient care and nurses' job satisfaction. (Our RN turnover rates were a major problem.) Surprisingly, we found that all of the improvements we made to reduce non-nursing activities had very little impact on the way nurses spent their time; most notably, the time thus freed up did not result in nurses spending more time with patients. This led us to begin looking more directly at the work of nursing, which ultimately resulted in a major redesign of the way nursing work in hospitals was conceptualized, defined, and delivered.

In looking at the actual work nurses were engaged in, expectations for a more comprehensive approach to practice were surfacing. However, the task-based work organization of team nursing was a fundamental barrier to creating a more comprehensive and professional focus on patient care. Consequently (and unknowingly), the intrusiveness of the project itself—of the reality of being studied and assessed and asked to make many changes in a short period of time—created enormous pressure on the nurses, affecting all levels of the staff. Although they were originally enthusiastic about the project, this new intense focus on their day-to-day work activities proved intolerable, and they rebelled. One day the staff announced they had decided as a whole to resign if the project wasn't stopped.

It is important to note that this unit was selected in the first place because of the excellent leadership of its nurse manager and because the staff was highly competent and had very high morale. This rebellion can be understood partly in the context of overall societal unrest at the time, combined with the ongoing pressure created by the project. Needless to say, this rebellion looked to most of us like a major catastrophe.

The clinical nursing director of the service and I decided to call an emergency meeting of the staff that evening at my home. Nearly all staff members from all different levels came. We sat around the fireplace and talked about what was going on and about the kind of care we really wanted patients on Unit 32 to be getting. The staff RNs asked if they could please not be "team leaders" the next day. The director and I reluctantly, and with full awareness of the risks we were taking, said yes. That "yes"—a "yes" that acknowledged that the people closest to the work were in the best position to decide how it should be done—was the beginning of Primary Nursing. It did not have a name, and it did not even have a structure on day one. The nurses reorganized the way things were done and the way patients were assigned. Keeping within appropriate and licensed scopes of responsibility for the various levels of staff, the reorganization of work took place in the best way possible, by the design of those highly qualified people. This was a true re-engineering of nursing care delivery.

In my capacity as co-director of the project, I had access to some of the finest minds at the University of Minnesota in the fields of sociology, philosophies of management, industrial relations, nursing theories, industrial engineering, and research into hospital administration. The next several months were a period of intense creative development. The entire staff, along with individuals from a broad spectrum of expertise, engaged in a conversation that led to the development of the delivery system called Primary Nursing.

The impact of the change was seen and felt almost immediately. The pace of the unit seemed to slow down almost miraculously. Nurses stayed in patient rooms for longer stretches of time, resulting in a dramatic shift in the energy of the unit. People asked me whether Unit 32 now had more staff because things seem so much calmer. Several physicians started asking to have all of their patients admitted to Unit 32. They didn't know why; they just knew things were working better.

The individuals who were available to help us think through the organizational implications were very active during this time. We were soon able to identify some fundamental principles of organizational changes that were occurring organically on the unit. Even though we didn't have the language to name it then, it was a change in focus from task-based to relationship-based practice. Eventually we understood that one historic "yes" resulted in the design of a new care delivery system. The principles of that system began to emerge from the quickly evolving daily practice of the staff nurses, coupled with the conceptual contributions of our expert advisors.

The principles identified all those years ago are still the fundamental structure of the delivery system of Primary Nursing as it is currently practiced throughout the world. The core concept of the RN taking full "responsibility, authority, and accountability" for his or her patients became the foundation of a movement that continues to progress throughout nursing and throughout other complex organizations.

As time went on, it became apparent that the two competing theories of management exemplified by team nursing and Primary Nursing could not exist simultaneously in a healthy system. For this reason, we made sure that transforming the authoritarianism of the traditional head nurse role was part of the immediate change process. It became clear that head nurses who were comfortable with an empowered staff could easily implement Primary Nursing, whereas those who needed to control their staff members' practice themselves had a very difficult time with it.

> *The core concept of the RN taking full "responsibility, authority, and accountability" for his or her patients became the foundation of a movement that continues to progress throughout nursing and throughout other complex organizations.*

Over the next ten years, my work involved changing the administrative structures within nursing departments from the command-and-control philosophy of the past to one of growth and development based on clarity of responsibility, delegation of commensurate authority, and nurses holding themselves accountable for the quality-of-care decisions they make.

Interestingly, just as we were developing Primary Nursing at the University of Minnesota Hospital, three other nurse leaders in four separate venues across the country simultaneously studied the idea of decentralization. It was during a conversation at a national conference that this convergence surfaced. During the late sixties, Joyce Clifford was teaching in a master's program in nursing administration at the University of Indiana. She taught her students about the theory of decentralization and its potential impact on the way nursing departments operated. Simultaneously, Janet Kraegle, Virginia Mousseau, and their colleagues were implementing the decentralized organization of supplies and care support materials, revising the physical characteristics of a unit to achieve a point-of-use supply distribution system. At the same time, Rosamunde Gabrielson implemented a decentralized administrative structure at what was then called Good Samaritan Hospital in Phoenix, Arizona. Decentralization was clearly an idea whose time had come.

And the Pendulum Continues to Swing ...

It's extremely important to remember that the adoption of Primary Nursing was the choice of the nurses who implemented it. Every previous care delivery system was created and implemented in response to changes in the culture and skill mix, without consideration of what would be best for patients and families or what sort of work culture would keep nurses physically and emotionally healthy. Primary Nursing wasn't owned by any leadership association or individual. It was organic, and this organic expression of nursing—one that safeguards the nurse–patient relationship—was replacing team nursing and functional nursing all over the country ... until another societal change came in the late 1980s and 1990s. This era was marked by increased patient acuity levels and decreases in hospital staffing, as well as technical and financial drivers, increased regulation, and the redesign of the health care system based on the capitalistic mindset. These factors drove us back toward the task-based practice and mindset that is all too prevalent today.

In this truly painful era, role differentiation and specialization were obliterated, and generic categories of health care workers were created. Work redesign projects purporting to streamline the work were actually thinly disguised changes in the skill mix designed to save salary dollars by reducing the numbers of RNs. That insidious trend was ironically termed "patient-centered care." The outcome was highly fragmented, task-based nursing that reduced morale and dispirited even the most dedicated nurses.

Not surprisingly, the 1990s left many nurses feeling overworked, underappreciated, and uninspired. "I love patient care," bedside staff nurses frequently said, "but I hate my job." However, as the 21st century started, nursing began once again to own its destiny. Extreme staffing shortages have forced a reidentification with the fundamental values of the profession, and society speaks loudly and clearly of its frustration with today's health care system, demanding humane treatment and identifying nurses as the purveyors of that treatment. Studies began demonstrating the impact of staffing and percentage of professional nurses on patient mortality and morbidity. Researchers such as Linda Aiken and Colleen Goode contributed important evidence that professional nursing impacted the quality and safety of patient care. Hospital administrators began to recognize the contribution of nursing to patient experience scores and core measures. The intense drive toward positive patient experience being led by the Centers for Medicare and Medicaid (CMS) has refocused attention on relationships and the impact of professional nurses. The Magnet® standards (instituted in the early 1990s), which require structural empowerment to achieve successful designation, have further driven decentralized decision making within nursing departments. These structures have given an additional boost to professional practice.

Nursing's Covenant with Society

As I look back at the long history of nursing, I've come to appreciate how constant nursing's covenant with society is, despite the phenomenal changes within society as a whole. Changes in the world forced us, as a profession, to alter many aspects of our practice. Technological advances have shortened hospitalizations. The Internet gave the public access to vast amounts of information formerly owned only by health care professionals. Health care is now a business. Nursing sought none of these changes; nevertheless, we own our response to them. As a profession, nursing has the right and responsibility to decide the amount, degree, and kind of nursing care we will deliver to patients within the constraints that society and health care systems set. As the profession matures, we as nurses are moving toward the understanding that, in the real world, it is our right and responsibility to deliver our services in a way that is consistent with our fundamental contract with society. There is a new courage among nurses, and it is translating into positive change.

The successful implementation of decentralization principles within a hospital bureaucracy means that, forevermore, the nursing profession knows it has a choice between task-based nursing care and relationship-based nursing care. We also know there are forces that impact the ease or difficulty of making that choice. The intense pressure of using complex data in a highly technical activity often drives the caregiver's attention away from the human dimension of the practice. The pendulum continues to swing: Continuity of care becomes more challenging due to shortened lengths of stay, coupled with 12-hour shifts; with financial concerns rather than patient acuity dictating skill mix; and with CEOs, CNOs, and COOs philosophically uncomfortable with giving direct care nurses authority over patient care. These factors and others challenge the sustained implementation of Primary Nursing.

Remember, however, that it is in the nature of a pendulum to swing back and forth almost equally. Although the pendulum seems to have swung from task-based nursing toward relationship-based nursing at this point in our history, there is always the risk (or perhaps even the inevitability) of people arriving on the scene who will try to cause it to swing back. It is my opinion that the predominant factor in moving the pendulum away from relationship-based practice in any organization is a change in administrative philosophy. New leaders seem to feel the need to generate a shift in the fundamental orientation of the institution. This need is often expressed by changing structures, moving people around in the top positions, letting a few people go, and cutting budgets to improve margins. Although it is possible that no injury to relationship-based practice is intended, these changes often do more to reduce the commitment to relationship-based practice than other factors. We see in the history of nursing, over and over, that in times of change, it is far less risky to just do the tasks—to do what can be measured and documented and therefore valued and rewarded.

While Primary Nursing may seem to some to be an unrealistic dream, the reality is that versions of it are thriving all around us. The principles of professional autonomous practice are continuously being re-envisioned, sometimes through the formation of new positions such as care coordinator and care manager. It doesn't matter what the role is called. What matters is that the patients and their families know the name of the nurse who is responsible for managing their care over time. If that is known, then the system is in place. It is all about the nurse–patient relationship.

Today, increasing numbers of courageous health care administrators are investing in transforming the cultures of their organizations to focus on relationships. They are reaping the benefits of engaged and committed employees and patients who experience personalized and compassionate care. Are you satisfied with this being only a temporary change—a mere trend we enjoy for a period of time, only to lose it when the next big wave of societal or professional change comes? Are you seeing the swing of the pendulum back to task-based practice as an inevitability? If so, remember this: It is also the nature of a pendulum to stop when an outside force stops it.

As this book goes to press, the pendulum is swinging toward relationship-based practice once again. Patients and families are demanding it, and thanks to superb resources like Koloroutis and Trout's *See Me as a Person: Creating Therapeutic Relationships with Patients and Their Families,* nurses and clinicians in all disciplines now have a blueprint for making authentic connections. Each time the pendulum returns to a relationship-based practice delivery system, patients receive the kind of coordinated and humane care they deserve. Isn't it time to reach out and stop the pendulum right where it is?

The future of nursing is in your hands.

Part II:

How to Implement Primary Nursing

We've had kids with severe, delicate diseases who had their lives saved because their Primary Nurse knew that if you don't keep a hat on them between the hours of 2:00 and 5:00 in the morning they're going to get radically hypothermic … And sometimes that's a child in protective custody, with no parents who will ever be at the bedside and no one else who will ever speak up for them.

NICOLE VANCE, BSN, RN
PRIMARY NURSE AT UC DAVIS MEDICAL CENTER

Chapter 2

Understanding Primary Nursing

And now that you don't have to be perfect, you can be good.

—John Steinbeck, *East of Eden*

There is universal agreement among nurses that their relationship with patients and patient families is a sacred and privileged trust (Koloroutis, 2004, p. 117). Primary Nursing is a care delivery system specifically designed to facilitate nurses in establishing, nurturing, and maximizing therapeutic relationships with their patients, thereby fulfilling this trust. It is the care delivery system that brings professional nursing practice to life. In this chapter we will deconstruct Primary Nursing in order to clarify its components, principles, infrastructure for design, and the process for leading the change from your current state to the desired state.

Before we go too far, however, we want to highlight three important and practical guidelines to inform your implementation process:

1. **Always make decisions in favor of the patient.** This guideline is built on the principle that the nurse's professional accountability is first and foremost to the patient. To achieve this guideline, ask questions such as:

   » In what ways does this decision serve the patient?

   » Is this in the best interest of the patient?

   » Will this decision most effectively contribute to the well-being and safe care of the patient?

» Will this decision fulfill my accountability to the patient?

These questions will guide you in determining what changes need to be put into place overall, what decisions need to look like in practice, and ultimately what the impact will be for the patients in your care.

2. **Never do anything that violates common sense.** If it makes no sense—even if it's "the way we've always done it"—don't do it. System design must never be allowed to violate common sense.

3. **Primary Nursing will always be imperfect.** However, if we hold the patient central and make decisions using our common sense, we will continuously improve in our ability to provide the best possible Primary Nursing care. Releasing the need to be perfect will allow you to move ahead with your implementation and continuously strive for improvement. Even though Primary Nursing cannot be perfect, it will provide patients with better care than they would receive in any other care delivery system.

With these guidelines in mind, we invite you to envision and personalize the ways you would want Primary Nursing brought to life in your practice setting. An important question to guide your thinking is: What would I want for myself or for my most beloved person in the world if either of us were sick and needed nursing care?

What is Primary Nursing?

Primary Nursing is a care delivery system designed (1) to allocate responsibility for each patient's care to one individual nurse for the duration of the patient's stay, visit, or series of visits and (2) to assign to this nurse the actual provision of the patient's care whenever possible. The Primary Nurse leaves information and instructions about that patient's care so that the associate nurses who provide direct care in the Primary Nurse's absence know about the patient as a person and exactly how care should be administered to this particular person. The Primary Nurse also accepts major responsibility for preparing the patient and family for discharge.

> Primary Nursing is not that different from what we already do every day, taking care of patients, building care plans, building relationships. The reasons people go into nursing is to make a difference, and Primary Nursing allows you to provide a different level of comfort. So many patients say, "Just seeing your face makes me feel more at ease."
>
> *—Kathleen Fowler, BSN, RN*
> *Primary Nurse at OSUCCC—James*

Primary Nursing is a system for delivering nursing care in any setting. It was developed on a real nursing unit in a real hospital during a serious nursing shortage. The nursing staff was not handpicked, nor were they considered unusually qualified. Thus, the system is designed for maximum use of available resources. No additional money was allocated during the development phase. Primary Nursing is an innovation that works in the real world because that is the crucible in which it was originally developed, tested, and refined.

High-quality nursing care—care that is individualized to a particular patient and administered compassionately, competently, and with continuity—should be the goal of every nurse, educator, and manager.

High-quality nursing care—care that is individualized to a particular patient and administered compassionately, competently, and with continuity—should be the goal of every nurse, educator, and manager. Primary Nursing is a proven way of achieving that quality of care. Even when Marie Manthey and her team began the formal practice of Primary Nursing in the late 1960s, it was not really a new idea. It is the most logical approach to caring for sick people in the way we would like to be cared for if we were sick. However, the process of returning to these simple, common-sense values was then, and still is, revolutionary in that it represents a reallocation of power from an authoritarian bureaucracy to the staff nurse who is responsible for the care of a sick person.

Primary Nursing is the care delivery system that best supports professional nursing practice. It focuses on the nurse–patient relationship, strengthens accountability for care, and facilitates patient and family involvement in the planning of care. The Primary Nurse and the patient are in a therapeutic partnership rather than a superior–subordinate relationship.

This care delivery system allows a Primary Nurse to establish a therapeutic relationship with each patient and family. The Primary RN initiates the relationship, which remains in effect for an episode of care or service (whether that episode spans a few hours or a number of days, weeks, or months). It is equally effective in ambulatory, inpatient, home care, and procedural departments.

Some defining components of Primary Nursing are as follows:

- Primary Nurses accept responsibility for decision making regarding the nursing care the patient receives during a health, illness, or procedural event.

- The Primary Nurse–patient relationship is known to the patient and family.

- Other members of the health care team honor and safeguard the Primary Nurse relationship.

It's important to realize that the Primary Nurse does not provide all patient care. In partnership with the patient, the RN identifies the patient's unique health needs and priorities, establishes an individualized plan of care, provides direct care as appropriate, and communicates the plan to other members of the team. LPNs or nursing assistants should be assigned to the RN rather than to the patient, to make clear that the RN is overseeing and/or directing the care.

Associate nurses provide direct care in the absence of the Primary Nurse. These individuals provide care based on the plan of care established by the Primary Nurse, changing it only when the patient's condition warrants a change and the Primary Nurse is not available. Associate nurses are assigned as consistently as possible to maximize continuity of care and reduce the number of caregivers the patient encounters.

Outcomes That Can be Expected in a Primary Nursing Care Delivery System

Over the past several decades, many organizations have adopted Primary Nursing as their nursing care delivery system. Several predictable outcomes have been enjoyed by people providing and receiving care in a Primary Nursing care delivery system. In well over four decades of Primary Nursing across the world, these are the most prevalent outcomes reported (Bond, Bond, Fowler, & Fall, 1991; Gardner, 1991; Gardner & Tilbury, 1991; Persky, Felgen, & Nelson, 2012; Rathert & May, 2007; Sellick, Russell, & Beckmann, 2003):

- Nurses achieve a new sense of autonomy and confidence in their ability to manage their patients' nursing care.

- Patients feel included in their care and feel seen as people, thereby experiencing greater feelings of trust and safety.

- Nurses experience greater professional satisfaction.

- Nurses gain new perspectives on teamwork and the interdependence of RNs with LPNs and NAs, leading to a higher level of professional nursing practice.

- Nursing staff experience higher levels of engagement and find new meaning and purpose in their work.

- Nurses and physicians experience enhanced collaboration and collegiality.

- Patients experience improved outcomes and fewer complications such as falls, infections, or readmissions.

- Patients perceive improved communication and pain control.

An Unwavering Commitment to Decentralized Decision Making

Our many years of experience in the field have given us a great deal of confidence in the integrity of systems designed and refined by the staff members who will use them. We have always believed that such systems provide an effective way to deliver high-quality care, and our long-held belief is now also supported by evidence. For this reason, our recommendations for implementing Primary Nursing focus resolutely on staff member involvement in the process.

The humanization of hospital care has been Marie's strongest motivation since the early 1960s and a passion of Susan's since becoming a Primary Nurse as a new graduate in 1975. Key to this humanization is the establishment of a partnership paradigm in which decision making is decentralized.

When decision making is *centralized*, it rests squarely with those at the top of the org chart, far from the point of care and service. A *decentralized* structure creates a culture of partnership within an organization, actively inviting the best thinking of the people closest to the work.

> Decentralized decision making creates an organizational culture within which teamwork can thrive, safety is maximized, and compassionate treatment of patients and families can most effectively be provided and maintained.

Decentralized decision making creates an organizational culture within which teamwork can thrive, safety is maximized, and compassionate treatment of patients and families can most effectively be provided and maintained. In order for patients to be treated as partners in their own care, the staff who deliver the care must be treated as respected, empowered partners by the management of the institution. Decentralized decision making creates an organizational structure wherein authority for decisions about care rests with the person closest to the work, in this case, the nurse. By authorizing the nurse who delivers care to decide how that care will be delivered, the institution acknowledges that staff nurses are intelligent, educated people who are capable of deciding how to provide sensitive and sensible individualized care. One of the fundamental principles of the partnership paradigm is that a commitment to partnership must be consistent. If partnership is selective or intermittent, care is not being delivered within a partnership paradigm. For this reason, one of the most effective ways to ensure that nurses will consistently partner with patients and their families is for managers to consistently partner with the staff.

Management responsibilities in a decentralized decision-making structure are different from those in a centralized, authoritarian structure. One of the most obvious differences is that the role of managers in a decentralized setting is as developers of people rather than as dictators of systems, processes, and actions. In Primary Nursing implementation, the change process is designed and led by the staff nurses. The ultimate decisions about how to put the Primary Nursing system into effect must be made at the staff nurse level. Otherwise, decentralized decision making has not been experienced by the staff nurses and will not become the norm for the clinical decision making required by the care delivery system.

The implementation process we recommend gives all staff members an opportunity to use the rights they have always possessed. Nurses need to develop an appreciation for the reality of their own authority. Many nurses have been made to feel that because physicians control medical treatment and hospital administrators define the mission and policies of the hospital, the people in these roles also have authority and control over all aspects of nursing practice. If nurse executives are to be held accountable for the quality of care administered by the nursing staff, they must have authority to set the standards of care and introduce appropriate delivery systems. This authority legitimately rests with CNOs by virtue of the responsibility they have accepted.

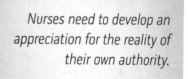

Nurses need to develop an appreciation for the reality of their own authority.

There is a call to action in that last paragraph. However, it is not a call for CNOs to "pull rank" on anyone else on any subject at any point. It's a call for nurse leaders at all levels to see themselves as inherent partners in the design and implementation of nursing and also as inherent partners in the design of care across disciplines in the organization as a whole. They know the work because they do (or have done) the work, and it is essential that their active partnership be sought by everyone charged with designing care in their organizations. The flip side of this call to action is for CNOs to see themselves as equal partners with physicians and hospital administrators and to step fully into their authority.

Years ago, CNOs used to ask Marie how she got the physicians or the hospital administrator to "let her" do Primary Nursing. The truth is Marie didn't ask them; she just did it. Since Primary Nursing usually does not cost any more money in salary dollars, permission from the hospital administrator is not necessary. However, in introducing the concept, it is extremely important that all key members of the institution are invited into partnership and offered a chance to understand fully the changes being made.

Relationship-Based Care

Relationship-Based Care (RBC) is a model for cultural transformation that has as one of its components the Primary Nursing care delivery system. (See Figure 2.1.) Relationship-Based Care identifies three crucial relationships for the provision of humane and compassionate health care. These three relationships are the caregiver's relationship with the patient/family, relationships among colleagues, and the caregiver's relationship with self (Koloroutis, 2004). It includes principles that shape caring behaviors, and these principles guide the transformation of infrastructure, processes, systems, and practices to support caregivers in all disciplines in creating therapeutic relationships with patients and families.

> I don't think I could be a nurse if we didn't have this relationship-based focus. I think the best part of nursing is having these relationships.
>
> —Heidi Nolen, BSN, RN
> Primary Nurse at UC Davis Medical Center

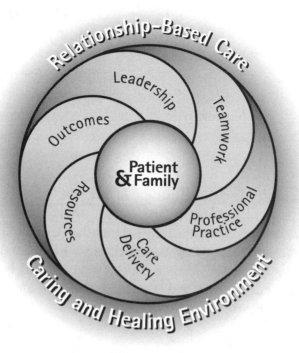

Figure 2.1: Relationship-Based Care Model

While Primary Nursing is essential in order for RBC to be expressed in its most effective form, Primary Nursing can be implemented in any department in any organization whether or not RBC is the organizational model. It is important to understand that the decision of what care delivery system to use can be determined at the local level. Because Primary Nursing requires no additional funds for personnel (assuming that staffing is adequate to begin with), the decision to implement it can be made by people at the point of care delivery. For the purposes of this book, however, we are focusing on organization-wide implementations in which a decision has been made to implement Primary Nursing as the care delivery system and the culture and systems are aligned to support it.

> *It is important to understand that the decision of what care delivery system to use can be determined at the local level.*

> The practice of Primary Nursing reinforces our belief that the relationships we build have the inherent capacity to promote health, healing, and wholeness.
>
> —*Carol Robinson, RN, MPA, NEA-BC, FAAN*
> *Chief Patient Care Services Officer and Director of Nursing,*
> *Primary Nurse and administrative champion of Primary Nursing since 1992*

The Four Elements That Define Care Delivery Systems

The care delivery system within Relationship-Based Care is Primary Nursing. A care delivery system is defined by four elements: (1) responsibility for relationships and decision making, (2) how work is allocated, (3) how communication occurs, and (4) management or leadership focus and philosophy. (See Figure 2.2.)

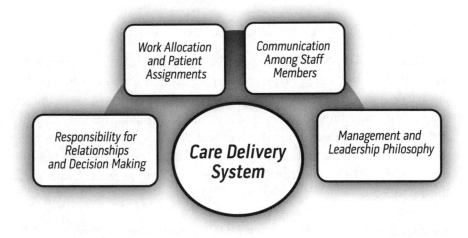

Figure 2.2: The Four Elements of a Care Delivery System

How these four defining elements are actualized ultimately determines how the care delivery system works and what it is. It sometimes happens that leaders in an organization think they are engaging in a particular care delivery system when it really is not. For example, if an organization says it is doing Primary Nursing, but responsibility for decision making is not given to the Primary Nurses, Primary Nursing is not happening. A care delivery system does not depend on skill mix, staffing patterns, or the amount of work required. It is how these four elements are defined and actualized that determines what sort of care delivery system is really in place.

We have descriptions below of how Primary Nursing is actualized through each of these elements. In Appendix A, we have provided a table that details how these elements are actualized for other care delivery systems, such as total patient care, team nursing, and functional nursing, in comparison to Primary Nursing.

The four definitions that follow apply to both inpatient and ambulatory settings. They should be adjusted to make sense for each setting, the types of patients treated, and the uniqueness of physical space, systems, and other factors specific to the area practicing Primary Nursing.

Responsibility for Relationships and Decision Making

The Primary Nurse is given and accepts the responsibility for management of the care of a group or caseload of patients. In this role, the Primary Nurse, in partnership with the patient and/or family, identifies the needs of the patient and has the authority to develop a plan of care for the patient. Other nursing caregivers (associate nurses) are obligated to follow the plan of care determined by the Primary Nurse. This leads to the greatest level of consistency and, subsequently, a higher quality of care and higher satisfaction for the patient. If the Primary Nurse is not present, and the patient's condition or situation warrants changes in the plan of care, updating the plan becomes the responsibility of the RN caring for the patient. The primary relationship may begin before the admission of the patient and exists during the length of stay in a department or for an entire episode of care in an ambulatory or home care setting. In a medical home, primary care clinic, provider's office, or other ambulatory setting, a primary relationship with nurses and professionals in other disciplines may exist over extended periods of time, allowing individuals and their consistent team of health care professionals to work toward the achievement of long-term lifestyle and health goals.

Work Allocation and Patient Assignments

Daily care assignments are patient-based rather than based on the tasks or geography of the unit. Care assignments are determined by the acuity of the patient, the skill of the caregiver, and a commitment to maximizing continuity of care. Even though workload distribution requires consideration of the numbers of patients in an assignment, numbers are not the determining factor. Continuity of the nurse–patient relationship is directly linked to higher patient satisfaction, safety, overall quality, and improved work flow for the nurse (Alpert, Goldman, Kilroy, & Pike, 1992). Continuity of the Primary Nurse–patient relationship should be consistently maintained yet may not mean that the Primary Nurse always provides hands-on care for the patient. This is one of the places where the guidelines of "always make decisions in favor of the patient" and "always use common sense" come into play. For example, when the Primary Nurse is returning from time off, he or she must assess and determine what best serves the patient. In the vast majority of cases, it will be best for the patient that the Primary Nurse resumes direct care. In a few cases, the Primary Nurse may determine that the associate nurse should continue direct care, with the Primary Nurse continuing to coordinate the plan of care. Whatever the decision, the Primary Nurse continues in the primary relationship with the patient. There are also infrequent situations in which the Primary Nurse determines that the patient would be better served by transferring the Primary Nurse relationship to another nurse. This is accomplished with thorough communication with the patient and family.

Communication Among Staff Members

The well-being of the patient and consistency of care depend on the information flow between the patient and family and their caregivers. The Primary Nurse provides information about the patient to assure that care is coordinated and consistent with the patient's unique needs. The Primary Nurse collaborates with all members of the health care team on behalf of the patient, including engaging in creative problem solving to resolve identified or potential issues. The Primary Nurse is particularly aware of points of transition in the patient's experience and assures that appropriate information is conveyed and solicited when necessary.

Management and Leadership Philosophy

Managers create the culture to support Primary Nursing and professional practice. These leaders maintain a clear focus on care and service to patients and families, particularly when other initiatives and demands threaten that focus. They are committed to the development of the clinical staff as autonomous decision makers and problem solvers. The manager clearly articulates expectations for care and teamwork that provide an atmosphere in which individual growth and healthy team relationships are the norms. The leader creates a caring and supportive culture for the staff members so that they are free to provide care and support for their patients. In short, the manager cares for the nurses so the nurses can care for the patients.

> Primary Nursing definitely helped us to keep the patients as the focus, where they always should be, while all of the other changes were going on.
>
> —*Kathleen Fowler, BSN, RN*
> *Primary Nurse at OSUCCC—James*

Care Delivery Systems Are Different from Care Delivery Models and Professional Practice Models

The terms "care delivery system" and "care delivery model" are often (and erroneously) used interchangeably.

Whereas a care delivery system focuses specifically on how peoples' roles and responsibilities are organized and managed, a care delivery model is broader. A care delivery model represents an overarching collection of elements that, operating together, describe the practice of nursing

Whereas a care delivery system focuses specifically on how peoples' roles and responsibilities are organized and managed, a care delivery model is broader.

in a given organization. Elements that may be included in a care delivery model include:

- A theoretical framework

- A care delivery system

- Staffing plans and budgets

- Guidelines about staffing mix and/or skill level

- Educational requirements

- Committee/council structure

- Leadership philosophy

- Specialized RN roles such as clinical nurse specialist, case manager, discharge nurse, etc.

You will notice that a care delivery system, such as Primary Nursing, is just one dimension of the care delivery model. A department of nursing often has broad descriptions of all the dimensions of their model. All of these components together describe how the department of nursing will function and how nursing care will be delivered and managed. If the organization also creates a schematic image of those elements, that image is referred to in the Magnet® world, as a professional practice model.

"Professional practice model" (PPM) is another term that is often misused when speaking of care delivery models and systems. This term refers only to the schematic image that conceptualizes how nurses practice, collaborate, communicate, and develop professionally to achieve the highest quality of patient care possible. A professional practice model is grounded in nursing research and theory and includes ethical, clinical, and professional standards. The image depicts all the components of the care delivery model. Development of a PPM is a requirement of the American Nurses Credentialing Center (ANCC) Magnet Recognition Program® and is the overarching conceptual framework for practice within nursing and in partnership with other professional disciplines (ANCC, 2008).

> Primary Nursing has helped define the unique contribution of the nurse in health care, particularly in the hospital setting.
>
> —*Joan Wessman, RN, MS, CENP*

Primary Nursing and the Six Professional Practice Roles

Mary Koloroutis has defined six roles that provide a lens through which the full scope of professional nursing practice can be viewed and articulated (Koloroutis, 2004). (See Figure 2.3.) These roles are actualized through the Primary Nurse's relationship with the patient and family. They are valuable in helping nurses understand the full scope of their role as Primary Nurses, as well as helping the nurse articulate what patients, families, and colleagues can expect from the care they give.

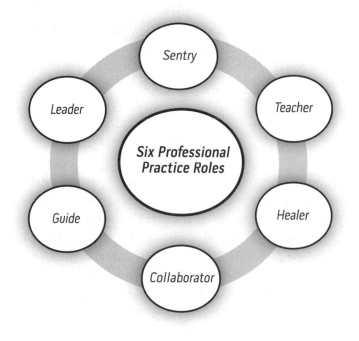

Figure 2.3: Six Professional Practice Roles
(Used with permission; Koloroutis, 2004)

Sentry

The Primary Nurse watches over the patient and family, benefiting from intentionally learning about the patient and family in a comprehensive manner. As sentry, the nurse assesses, monitors, and intervenes on behalf of the patient to prevent complications, promote healing, and optimize safe outcomes. The Primary Nurse owns the responsibility for overseeing and protecting.

> When the patient and family have a Primary Nurse, they have an advocate and they have someone to help them be their own advocate.
>
> —Heidi Nolen, BSN, RN
> Primary Nurse at UC Davis Medical Center

Teacher

The Primary Nurse ensures that the teaching provided takes into consideration not just the knowledge the health care team wants to impart but the knowledge the patient and family want and are ready to receive. The nurse maximizes the patients' and families' capacity to safely care for themselves and optimize their own well-being.

Healer

The Primary Nurse in the role of healer ensures that healing is approached holistically. The nurse establishes a therapeutic relationship with the patient and family. Even though the physical body may be the focus of the care experience, the plan of care includes attention to all aspects of the person's being—physical, spiritual, mental, and emotional. The plan addresses the meaning that patients and their families give to the illness or other health care situation and its implications for their lives. Nursing interventions are based on initial and ongoing assessments to meet all the individual's needs—body, mind, and spirit.

Collaborator

The Primary Nurse works in partnership with all members of the health care team as well as the patient and family. The Primary Nurse coordinates care, ensuring that the interprofessional team is working cooperatively in the best interest of the patient.

Guide

The Primary Nurse develops a plan to ensure that the patient and family receive the information needed to navigate their health care experience. The amount and degree of information provided depend on the current situation the patient and family are experiencing. For example, early in a post-surgical course, the need may be to understand pain management. Later, a larger-scale plan may include the course of rehabilitation from hospital to home to the person's return to normal activity. In the role of guide, the Primary Nurse makes certain that the patient and family can function as full partners in care by ensuring that they have the information necessary to make decisions about their care.

Leader

The Primary Nurse as leader assumes the responsibility and ownership for ensuring that the care team is working as a team in the best interest of the patient. The RN advocates for and speaks on behalf of the patient when the patient is not able to do so (Koloroutis, 2004, pp. 129–131; adapted with permission).

Summary of Key Points

- Primary Nursing is a delivery system specifically designed to facilitate nurses in establishing, nurturing, and maximizing therapeutic relationships with their patients.

- Three guidelines inform the successful implementation of Primary Nursing:

1. Always make decisions in favor of the patient.

2. Never do anything that violates common sense.

3. Primary Nursing will always be imperfect.

- Primary Nursing is a system for delivering nursing care in any setting, is highly customized to suit the needs of individual patient populations and teams, and is designed through a shared vision.

- The Primary Nurse accepts responsibility for the nursing care of a patient during the person's episode of care on a particular unit, department, outpatient clinic, or in home care.

- Primary Nursing works in the real world because it was designed and tested by clinical nurses to improve their care for patients and families; the decisions for how Primary Nursing is implemented must be made at the staff nurse level.

- The Primary Nurse is known by name to the patient, the family, and the other members of the health care team.

- Patient outcomes include greater patient involvement and coordination of care, higher satisfaction with care, improved clinical outcomes, and fewer complications such as falls, infections, or readmission.

- Primary Nurses experience higher autonomy and confidence in their ability to coordinate care, higher levels of engagement, a greater sense of meaning and purpose in their work, and improved communication/collaboration with physicians and other members of the team.

- Relationship-Based Care is an organizational model that has the Primary Nursing care delivery system as a core dimension.

- A care delivery system is not a care delivery model.

  » A care delivery model focuses on how people's roles and responsibilities are organized and managed.

» A care delivery system is one part of a broader care delivery model and is defined by four elements:

1. Responsibility for relationships and decision making

2. Work allocation and patient assignments

3. Communication among staff members

4. Management and leadership philosophy

- A professional practice model (PPM) conceptualizes how nurses practice, collaborate, and develop professionally to achieve the highest quality of patient care. A professional practice model is grounded in nursing research and theory and includes ethical, clinical, and professional standards.

- Six practice roles provide a lens to understand and articulate the professional scope of nursing practice and can be actualized through the Primary Nurse role:

1. Sentry

2. Teacher

3. Healer

4. Collaborator

5. Guide

6. Leader

Questions for Reflection

- What would you want in a relationship with a Primary Nurse if you needed care or if the person you love most in this world needed care? What would matter most?

- What do you think contributes to the improved outcomes when patients are cared for in a Primary Nursing care delivery system?

- Consider the three guidelines for implementing Primary Nursing: (1) Always make decisions in favor of the patient. (2) Never violate common sense. (3) Primary Nursing will always be imperfect. What do these guidelines mean to you? What are some specific ways you can apply them to help move your implementation plan forward?

- What is your understanding of what it takes to be in a therapeutic relationship? What are some ways in which you and your colleagues can support one another in gaining greater proficiency in this key relationship?

- What structures currently support the therapeutic relationship with your patient and families (e.g., change-of-shift report involving the patient/family, one-on-one time with the patient/family/nurse every shift, interdisciplinary collaboration/rounds, other)? What structures may need to be changed?

- What does the role of sentry mean to you? How is that role brought to life in your care of a patient/family?

I have never experienced another system where nurses were so committed to the quality of life of the patients and their families.

JUNE WERNER, MN, MSN, RN, CNAA
PRIMARY NURSING PIONEER

Chapter 3

Preparing for Implementation:
Leading Lasting Change

There is an effective formula for leading the deep and lasting change to Primary Nursing that will assist leaders in both organizing the change and being comprehensive in the design and implementation of it. This formula, known as I_2E_2, includes four phases that cycle and repeat as the change moves forward (Felgen, 2007). The four elements in this simple formula are (1) Inspiration, (2) Infrastructure, (3) Education, and (4) Evidence. (See Figure 3.1.) Once a vision for practice becomes clear, you must make sure that the team stays inspired (I_1), ensure that the infrastructure (I_2) supports the vision, provide all the necessary education (E_1), and decide what evidence (E_2) (outcomes) will help to show that your vision has been achieved. When you address all of these elements systematically as the implementation progresses, change can be both comprehensive and sustainable.

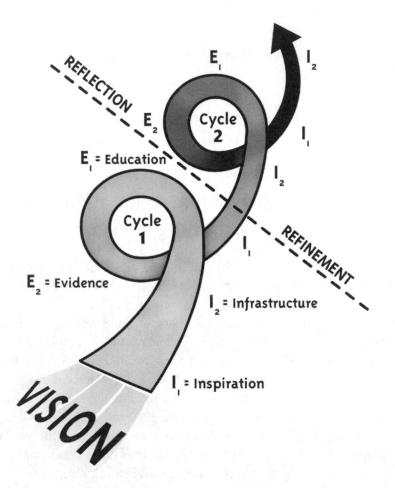

Figure 3.1: Jayne Felgen's I_2E_2 Model

The implementation of Primary Nursing will require much testing of new ideas. As ideas are tested, they may be found to work well, or it may be discovered that something is lacking. The systematic use of I_2E_2 will help identify, for example, whether a new idea needs additional educational support or an infrastructural change is necessary in order to make the desired behavior a path of least resistance for the people involved. It may also help to identify an "inspiration deficit" around a proposed change, meaning that people aren't clear on the meaning, purpose, or advantages of the change. I_2E_2 provides a framework through which you can look methodically and strategically at any organizational change undertaken in support of implementing Primary Nursing.

> With any sort of change, it takes a long time to be successful, to get into the habit, into the new routine, getting people involved, and tracking your progress. I use the I_2E_2 model. This is one of the first projects where we used I_2E_2, which I think is great. I was able to track our progress, and it's easy to share with other units, "These are the steps we took to do it ..."
>
> —*Kathleen Fowler, BSN, RN*
> *Primary Nurse at OSUCCC—James*

Lasting Change Begins with a Clear Vision

All satisfying, long-lasting changes start with a clear vision. In this case, you will want to create a personal vision and a shared vision for what Primary Nursing will look like in the department and the organization. You must have an image of the desired future in concrete and measurable terms. Felgen provides the following guidance for creating your vision:

- Construct your vision with its end use in mind.

- Use it as a touchstone for all that you do.

- Make the vision live in the daily practices in your work area.

- Write your vision statement in the present tense as though it is already happening. This helps generate a clear and tangible direction and inspires people to bring it to life. (Felgen, 2007)

Application: Creating Your Vision of Primary Nursing

As you think about your vision for Primary Nursing, it will be helpful for you to reflect on what you would want for yourself or a loved one receiving nursing care. Consider the care experience you hope to have in any possible setting: acute care; an emergency department; a primary care office; before, during, and after a procedure or surgery; and so on. As you reflect, think about how your care would be enhanced if one nurse took responsibility for:

- Knowing you, finding out what is most important to you during your episode of care/illness.

- Understanding what this experience means to you.

- Developing a plan for care that honors your preferences.

- Communicating your preferences, concerns, and goals to other members of the health care team.

- Providing your daily care whenever possible.

- Managing your discharge care needs.

The Components of the I_2E_2 Model Defined

Inspiration

Lasting change will occur only if we touch the core values and imagination of all those who are expected to implement change in a system. When desired changes include individual dreams and visions, and a collective vision is clearly linked with personal and organizational purpose and values, hope emerges that these changes will make a difference. Inspiration then becomes a driving force.

The inspiration element of the model answers these questions:

- How will this change improve the experience of our patients and their families?

- What good things are already happening that we can use as sources of inspiration?

- What inspires us most about this vision for change?

- What will sustain our inspiration so that we can move forward?

- How can we inspire and energize others to work toward this vision?

Application of Inspiration to Primary Nursing

Generating inspiration is a critical component of your plan to implement Primary Nursing. Consider whether you have existing practices you can use for inspiration or if you need to develop new or additional strategies. Here are some classic strategies you might consider for keeping yourself and others inspired:

- In small groups, share stories of a time when your deep relationship with a patient or family made a positive difference in their care—a time when you felt a special connection.

- Reflect upon what drew you into health care; have a small group of co-workers describe why they entered the nursing profession and what gives them the most joy in their work.

- Have a meaningful conversation with patients who had a Primary Nurse. Find out what that relationship meant to them. Collect and share these insights with the entire unit.

- Discuss the professional satisfaction enjoyed when you or your peers practiced Primary Nursing in the past.

- Explore ways to share inspirational thoughts or sayings during each shift; perhaps at huddles or as you begin your day.

At each unit council meeting I go over our audits and updates. I send out emails with our updates, because not everyone can attend the meeting, and I think the audit reports make people want to do better. I think when they see a number, they want to do the best they can. If they see that what they're doing is working, and they see where they need to improve, that really makes a big difference as well. I always point out what's going well, and *then* the things to work on. I like to focus on the positive.

—*Kathleen Fowler, BSN, RN*
Primary Nurse at OSUCCC—James

Infrastructure

Successful change establishes new practices, systems, and processes through which the collective vision is achieved and sustained. Changes to infrastructure must occur at three levels of the organization or department:

1. **Strategic**: Mission, vision, and goals (culture of the organization or department).

2. **Operational**: Roles, responsibilities, standards, policies, reporting structures, financial and information systems (departments across the organization).

3. **Tactical**: Daily practices, routines, and standards (at the individual level—at the point of care and service).

Leaders must intentionally weave elements of the change into the organization's fabric at every level.

Application of Infrastructure to Primary Nursing

No amount of good intentions will establish Primary Nursing as your care delivery system if the systems, processes, and physical setup of your department do not actively support it. Changes will likely be necessary. If you desire behavioral changes, adjusting your infrastructure in ways that make those new behaviors a path of least resistance will help bring those changes to life. Consider not only what barriers to the desired behaviors you can remove but also what you can change in order to actively encourage the desired behaviors.

> *Successful change establishes new practices, systems, and processes through which the collective vision is achieved and sustained.*

Your first step in designing an infrastructure that will bring Primary Nursing to life is to create a staff council or unit practice council (UPC).

(UPCs will be discussed at length in Chapter 4.) The second step is the actual building of the plan for implementation. This is a detailed action plan containing all of the decisions about what Primary Nursing will mean in your department and what new systems and processes will be required to help achieve your department's vision. Later in this book, you'll be given the tools to help you generate that plan.

Here are just a few examples of the decisions you will make about the infrastructure for Primary Nursing that will be unique for your department:

- Responsibilities of the Primary Nurse (PN) in your setting.

- Time from admission, or entry into your care setting, within which a PN is to be assigned.

- Criteria for who shall be PNs.

- Guidelines for how the PN is introduced to patient and family.

- Communication of the PN relationship to other health care team members.

- Where the name of the PN is written—in patient's room or chart and in a place visible to charge nurse, physicians, and other caregivers.

- How to ensure having the same PN in subsequent episodes of care.

- How the medical record shall reflect the PN role and care decisions.

- How the medical record shall reflect what the PN has learned about the patient as a person, as well as his or her needs.

- The role of associate nurses: responsibilities, how many, and so on.

- Situations in which the PN may transfer the PN role to another nurse.

Education

Education includes the knowledge, skill, and attitude development of all stakeholder groups involved in implementing the collective vision. The required education must be integrated into development plans for current and future employees and will likely necessitate development in all competency domains: clinical/technical, critical/creative thinking, intra-/ interpersonal, and leadership.

Application of Education to Primary Nursing

As you consider the education needed, be sure all the necessary components of education are included.

- Provide a definition of Primary Nursing.

- Describe the four components of a care delivery system, defining the differences between Primary Nursing, team nursing, functional nursing, and total patient care. (See Appendix A.)

- Ensure that the term "responsibility relationship" is understood. The Primary Nurse is responsible for establishing a therapeutic relationship and for partnering with the patient to develop the plan of care. Thereafter, all nurses caring for the patient/family are responsible for following the established plan and adjusting it in the absence of the Primary Nurse only when the patient's condition warrants a change.

- Educate every team member on your comprehensive plan for Primary Nursing, including all the infrastructure decisions you have made.

- Allow demonstrations and return demonstrations on how nurses introduce themselves and the role of Primary Nurse.

An introduction might sound something like:

Hello, my name is _____, and I will be your Primary Nurse. That means I'll coordinate your care while you're here. Together you and I will decide how your care will be provided and develop your plan of care. I'll find out what I need to know about you and your family in order to provide you with the best care. I'll make sure that others caring for you know what you and I have decided. I will usually provide your care when I am working. If something occurs that prevents me from doing this, I'll stop in and see how you're doing. I'll also make sure you have what you need before you go home.

Evidence

Measurement of the impact of change initiatives must drive day-to-day work and assume priority status in organizational or departmental leadership meetings and progress reports. The purpose of collecting and sharing evidence is to inspire greater commitment to the changes that have proven successful and to help redouble commitment to improving what has not yet demonstrated success. Evidence makes visible the degree to which behaviors are aligned with the overall vision.

Application of Evidence to Primary Nursing

Evidence of the success of Primary Nursing will be looked at from several perspectives. To begin with, you will want to consider evidence that ensures that Primary Nursing is indeed occurring. It is not enough to know that an individual has been assigned as a Primary Nurse; the relationship must be known to the patient, the family, and the other members of the health care team. In addition, you need to collect evidence that the responsibility relationship is making a difference for the patient and family.

Choose a few measures that are important to you. Here are some measures to consider:

- Patients know the name of their Primary Nurse. (This is an essential measurement.)

- Patients state that they feel seen as a person, safe, cared for, and/or included in the planning of the care they received. (Questions used to gather this information need to be evaluated for reliability.)

- Patient outcomes such as pain control, falls, and infections, etc.

- Length of stay, readmission rates, and/or frequency of visits.

- Patients demonstrate active responsibility in meeting their health care goals and take an active role in their follow-up visits.

Additionally, you will need to evaluate the impact of Primary Nursing on your co-workers. Is there improved teamwork, collaboration, and/or collegiality? You will need to determine whether current surveys provide the information you need. You may have to develop your own method of evaluation to generate evidence that will be the most meaningful to everyone involved.

> Some patients are still confused about who their Primary Nurse is. They think their Primary Nurse is the one assigned to them that day. Once you state the question more clearly, "Who's the nurse who is assigned to you all the time? Who's your advocate?" Then they remember and say, "She's Great!!" These are newly diagnosed leukemia patients and most have never been in a hospital. It's comforting for them, in this setting where everything is new and constantly changing, to know that they have someone who is consistently there for them.
>
> —*Kirsten Roblee, BSN, RN, OCN*
> *Primary Nurse at OSUCCC—James*

Before you implement Primary Nursing, it is necessary for the entire staff to have a clear understanding of:

1. What Primary Nursing is.

2. The importance of decentralized decision making.

3. The four elements of a care delivery system (see page 38).

4. How the I_2E_2 formula for sustainable change applies to your implementation of Primary Nursing.

The following chapters will guide you in making the needed decisions for a successful implementation.

Summary of Key Points

- I_2E_2 (Felgen, 2007) is a simple formula for leading any deep and lasting change. It has proven effective for implementing Primary Nursing.

- When all four elements of the I_2E_2 formula (inspiration, infrastructure, education, and evidence) are carefully implemented based on a shared vision, change will be both comprehensive and embedded in the practice culture.

- Develop your vision for Primary Nursing by reflecting on what you would want if you were a patient and how care would look if one nurse accepted clear responsibility for the patient and family.

- Inspiration is a driving force for change and is generated by touching the core values and imagination of all those who are expected to implement a change. Inspiration answers the question: Why is this change worthwhile to me?

- Classic strategies for inspiring self and others include storytelling and reflection about caring for patients, satisfying experiences as a nurse, listening and learning from patients and families, connecting to professional standards and code of ethics, as well as using inspirational quotes.

- No amount of good intentions will establish Primary Nursing as your care delivery system if the systems, processes, and physical setup (infrastructure) of your department do not actively support it.

- Your first step toward designing an infrastructure to bring Primary Nursing to life is to create a staff council or unit practice council (UPC). The second step is the actual building of the plan for implementation.

- Education includes knowledge, skill, and attitude development for all stakeholder groups involved in implementing the collective vision.

- The purpose of collecting and sharing evidence is to inspire greater commitment to the changes that have proven successful and to help redouble commitment to improving what has not yet demonstrated success.

Questions for Reflection

- What most inspires you about transforming your current care delivery system to a Primary Nursing care delivery system?

- How could we inspire and excite others about the potential impact of Primary Nursing on us and on our patients and families?

- What knowledge and skills would you want to develop further in order to fulfill your vision for Primary Nursing?

- What in your setting currently supports a Primary Nursing care delivery system?

- What needs to be changed or improved to support the change to Primary Nursing?

- What two to three measures would tell you that you are successfully transforming your care delivery system?

NOTES

Trust that it will work. Just be patient and give it time.

HEIDI NOLEN, BSN, RN
PRIMARY NURSE AT UC DAVIS MEDICAL CENTER

Chapter 4

The Role of the Unit Practice Council in Designing and Implementing Primary Nursing

Two groups of leaders will play key roles in ushering Primary Nursing into your department. The unit practice council (UPC) will design practice on your unit. It will include first-line staff members representing all roles and shifts from your department. All decisions about how Primary Nursing will look at the department level are made by this group. At the organizational level, a group of leaders who have a depth of experience in Primary Nursing will form a Primary Nursing coordinating committee, which will help the UPCs stay true to the principles of Primary Nursing as they customize it to their unique departments. This chapter will focus primarily on the work of the UPCs in designing, planning, and implementing Primary Nursing.

How Practice is Designed at the Unit Level and Overseen at the Organizational Level

Unit Practice Councils

As mentioned briefly in Chapter 3, unit-level staff councils are usually called unit practice councils (UPCs), but it is the concept, rather than the label you choose, that matters.

It's absolutely essential for UPCs to be clear about their responsibilities and level of authority for decision making. The members also need foundational education on core skills for running councils effectively. Start-up education should inspire them about their potential impact and should include content on:

- council responsibilities and scope

- levels of authority

- leadership roles

- leading an effective meeting

- communicating with all their peers

- taking minutes

- decision-making methods

- leading change

- systems of accountability (Wessel, 2012)

The council should include representatives of all of the roles in the department and should have sufficient membership to facilitate communication with all their peers between meetings through a communication network. Council membership comprising 15%–20% of the entire staff is ideal.

The manager should serve as an advisor and coach to members, being present for a part of each meeting, but the manager should not lead the council. It is essential that staff members are trusted to make the best decisions. (For more on the manager's role in UPCs, see Appendix B.)

Implementing Primary Nursing is accomplished largely through UPCs. Council members are given time for meetings as well as coaching to develop an action plan for their department on how they will implement the principles of Primary Nursing. This work gets to the heart of why many nurses went into health care. Council members make decisions that help them move away from a focus on tasks to a focus on professional practice and compassionate care. In addition to relationships with patients and families, Primary Nursing also focuses on smooth communication and collaboration with team members. UPCs plan innovative changes to strengthen teamwork and open communication.

The rest of this chapter assumes that your council of first-line caregivers is formed and well organized. Before you begin creating an action plan, you should have the components shown in Figure 4.1 solidly in place.

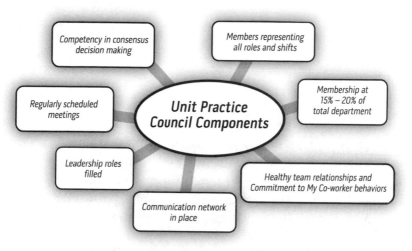

Figure 4.1: Unit Practice Council Components

Primary Nursing Coordinating Committee

When Primary Nursing is implemented as a directive from the organization, an organization-wide coordinating committee is formed to provide oversight. Members of this group will typically have prior experience with Primary Nursing and will act as both champions and mentors of the UPCs during implementation. Responsibilities of the Primary Nursing coordinating committee include:

- Educating and preparing the UPCs for their work in designing the details of Primary Nursing for their respective departments.

- Having council chair and/or co-chairs and their managers report progress several times during planning (this creates both support and an accountability loop).

- Designing methods to measure organization-wide outcomes and impact.

- Hearing the final action plans as presented by each council and manager.

- Tracking progress and outcomes.

- Guiding the councils in continuously sustaining and improving Primary Nursing.

Planning

When the unit practice council has met the criteria identified in Figure 4.1, they are ready to proceed to the planning phase of Primary Nursing implementation. Three to four months for planning is ideal, with regular meetings, perhaps twice per month. The work focuses on making decisions about how to translate the principles of Primary Nursing into a department-specific plan and on obtaining input from all co-workers every step of the way before making final decisions. (See Figure 4.2.)

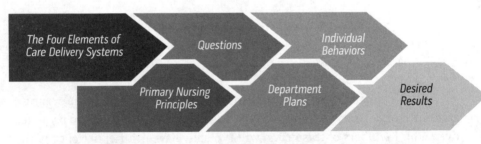

Figure 4.2: Building Blocks of Primary Nursing Implementation

When anybody's developing Primary Nursing, they need to customize it to their unit. Every unit works differently, and I think if you can make it your own, you're more likely to really do it and for it to work and for it to be sustainable.

—*Kathleen Fowler, BSN, RN*
Primary Nurse at OSUCCC—James

Principles of Primary Nursing to Guide Your Planning

The guiding framework for the plan to be developed by the UPC is a set of Primary Nursing principles. These principles are organized under the four elements introduced in Chapter 2:

- Responsibility for relationship and decision making.

- Work allocation and patient assignments.

- Communication with the health care team.

- Management and leadership philosophy.

A comprehensive set of worksheets is located in Appendix C to help you focus the work of the UPC and facilitate decision making about the elements of the care delivery system. This is accomplished through a set of questions carefully constructed for each set of principles. The questions that are applicable to your department should be viewed as a framework for discussion and decision making. If any questions are not applicable to your department, skip them and proceed to the next question.

After you're well versed in both the spirit and letter of the four elements of care delivery systems and the Primary Nursing principles, you'll begin customizing Primary Nursing to your unit using the questions in Appendix C. It is likely that through this process you'll learn as much about the functioning of your unit and all of its inhabitants as you will about Primary Nursing itself.

A few examples of the questions in Appendix C are included in this chapter for illustration purposes. UPC members should use the appendix as the agenda for their planning meetings. As the council members answer the questions that apply to them, the implementation plan emerges. It is absolutely essential that the council obtains input from all of their colleagues on all key decisions so that the ultimate plan represents the best thinking and solicits the active involvement of the entire department. Ownership and commitment to the new care delivery system are dependent upon active involvement by all members of the team. Without active involvement, people tend to remain detached or passive and think the change applies to "someone else."

We've integrated our pre-op, OR, and post-op into our Unit Practice Council. We have two representatives from each area, and we also invited people from among our patient care associates, our unit clerk, our orderly in the OR, some of our technical positions. That's why we have representation from all areas, which really helped in our council because we get a broad spectrum of ideas. What works for the OR won't necessarily work for another area. That diversity helped.

—Jane Czekajewski, BSN, RN, CNOR
Primary Nurse at OSUCCC—James

Excerpts from the Worksheet for Primary Nursing Implementation Plan (Appendix C)

Element 1: Responsibility for Relationship and Decision Making. One registered nurse accepts responsibility, authority, and accountability for managing the nursing care of specific patients.

Principles

1. One registered nurse (the Primary Nurse) develops a therapeutic relationship and individualized plan of care with the patient and family for their episode of care or service.

2. The patient and family are able to identify their Primary Nurse by name and understand that she or he is responsible for planning and coordinating their care.

3. Registered nurses are accountable for making decisions about the patient's care and for delivering or delegating activities of care and for effectively communicating those decisions to others, assuring smooth handoffs.

4. Other nurses caring for the patient in the absence of the Primary Nurse are responsible for following the plan of care developed by the Primary Nurse or to revise it based on the patient's response and changing needs.

5. Nursing roles are designed to fulfill the scope of practice statements in the state's Nurse Practice Act and to carry out their professional responsibilities.

Questions

What is the nature of the Primary Nurse relationship?

- What kinds of questions will the Primary Nurse use to begin to know the patient as a person?

- What will facilitate the Primary Nurse's ability to be present and attuned to the patient and family?

- Does education on therapeutic relationships need to be provided? If so, who will be responsible for providing education? How will you know when nurses understand this relationship?

- How will what is learned about the patient as a person (and his or her preferences) be communicated to the next caregiver?

What will it mean to be responsible for managing a patient's care for their entire episode of care?

- In what ways will Primary Nurses demonstrate their responsibilities for managing care for their Primary Patients in this department?

- When can other nurses make decisions regarding the patient's plan of care (POC)?

- How will these POC changes be communicated to the Primary Nurse?

Questions
Who will serve as Primary Nurses in this department? • Will all RNs be eligible to be a Primary Nurse? If not, what factors would exclude an RN from participating in this role? • How will supplemental, float, or PRN staff members be assigned? Under what circumstances? See Appendix C for the full list of questions.

Element 2: Work Allocation and Patient Assignments. The registered nurse has full authority for determining the kind and amount of nursing care a patient will receive and who will deliver that care.

Principles

1. Patient assignments are based on continuity of relationships, the complexity of care required, and the skills and knowledge of the caregiver.

2. Registered nurses have the authority for determining the kind and amount of nursing care a patient will receive, the work that care requires, how much of that work requires the expertise and time of the registered nurse, and how much can be delegated to other caregivers.

Questions
How will assignments be made to support Primary Nursing and continuity of relationships?

- How should the following considerations be prioritized for making shift/clinic assignments: prior relationship with the patient or family, skill/knowledge of the nurse/caregiver, patient acuity/safety, workload, room location? (Add other factors as appropriate.)

- What changes could be made to make continuity of assignments the norm?

- How will educational opportunities be provided for the growth and development of newer staff when preparing to be Primary Nurses (e.g., precepting, mentoring)?

- How will we ensure that staff schedules reflect a healthy balance of a patient-centric focus and self-care considerations?

See Appendix C for the full list of questions.

I know something that charge nurses will do, especially our assistant managers, is every so often they'll scan through the EMR and see that 10 patients on this floor don't have Primary Nurses yet, and even though it's because 6 of them came in last night, that's 10 patients too many. They'll just start having conversations with the bedside nurses, "What do you think? Is this somebody you could Primary? If not, why not?" They just help people to work through some of those things.

—*Nicole Vance, BSN, RN*
Primary Nurse at UC Davis Medical Center

Element 3: Communication with the Health Care Team. The registered nurse coordinates communication between the patient and family and members of the interdisciplinary team.

Principles

1. The Primary Nurse proactively seeks information and provides information to others involved in the care of the patient and family.

2. The Primary Nurse coordinates communication between the patient and family and other members of the interdisciplinary team.

3. As the nurse–patient relationship is established, the insight gained into what matters most to specific patients is communicated to other members of the team in order to ensure that the patient's care needs and preferences are met.

Questions
What systems will the Primary Nurse use to communicate and coordinate the nursing plan of care with other members of the nursing team and with physicians and people in other disciplines?

- How will the Primary Nurse communicate patient preferences and care decisions to other team members about the patient?

- How can the Primary Nurse efficiently gather information and suggestions about the patient from other team members?

- How can the patient and family be kept in the communication loop, receiving timely and consistent information about the plan of care and upcoming activities?

- What structure is or will be in place to ensure that the patient and family are able to contribute information, especially in the absence of the Primary Nurse? How will the structure be communicated to the patient/family?

Questions
What processes are in place to ensure communication between patient visits? • What guidelines exist or need to be developed to ensure that vital information is recorded for follow-up on the next visit? • How do people in different disciplines communicate during a visit and at subsequent patient encounters? See Appendix C for the full list of questions.

When we first decided to do Primary Nursing, we didn't know how to do report. We weren't really getting report from each other in a way that was helping us to get to know the patient. The OR nurse would run into the pre-op, look at the chart, hope it was all there, and the only time you'd talk to the pre-op nurse was if something was wrong. That wouldn't be enough connection if the pre-op nurse was the Primary Nurse, so we created this Pre-op to OR Handoff communication tool. Basically the pre-op nurse and the OR nurse go through the communication handoff tool in front of the patient. We tell the patient, "We're going to go over your plan of care in front of you. Please let us know if there's anything additional, if there's anything that we left out, or if you have any concerns." That really helps with our patients' satisfaction more than just handoff because we really get to know the patient, and their family is better informed and can be partners. It takes 5 minutes or less.

—*Jane Czekajewski, BSN, RN, CNOR*
Primary Nurse at OSUCCC–James

Element 4: Leadership and Management. The manager creates an environment that inspires healthy team relationships, professional nursing practice, and the provision of competent and compassionate care.

Principles

1. Managers articulate expectations for an environment in which healthy relationships thrive.

2. The manager promotes professional nursing practice in which registered nurses are autonomous decision makers and creative, empowered problem solvers.

3. The manager leads by inspiring, listening, coaching, and mentoring staff members to promote their professional growth and development.

Questions
Note: The manager should be invited to attend the council meeting in which these questions are discussed.

How will the manager and staff create a shared vision for Primary Nursing in this department?

- How will we create a vision that expresses what the patient will experience in a Primary Nurse relationship?

- What does the council imagine for nurses as they experience this role? What will nurses experience as they take ownership for planning care that is truly personalized?

- How can this vision be used to guide the development of the implementation plan?

- How can this vision be used to help educate all staff about the potential of Primary Nursing?

- How will this vision be described in practical ways?

Questions

How can positive caring relationships and collaboration be strengthened?

- What are the standards for how care team members treat each other in this department?

- How will we ensure that everyone follows these standards?

- What education and skill building are needed to build collaboration and effective conflict resolution among all team members?

See Appendix C for the full list of questions.

Summary of Plan to Implement Principles

The answers to all worksheet questions, discussed by the UPC with the input of the entire staff, will form the basis for your plan for implementing Primary Nursing. Here are just a few examples of the decisions you will have made about the infrastructure for Primary Nursing that will be unique for your department. They are the same items referred to in the previous chapter under a discussion of what items would comprise the Infrastructure element of your proposed change:

- Responsibilities of the Primary Nurse (PN) in your setting.

- Time from admission, or entry into your care setting, within which a PN is to be assigned.

- Criteria for who shall be PNs.

- Guidelines for how the Primary Nurse is introduced to patient and family.

- Communication of the PN relationship to other health care team members.

- Where the name of the PN is written—in patient's room or chart and in a place visible to charge nurse, physicians, and other caregivers.

- How to ensure having the same PN in subsequent episodes of care.

- How the medical record shall reflect the PN role and care decisions.

- How the medical record shall reflect what the PN has learned about the patient as a person, as well as his or her needs.

- The role of associate nurses: responsibilities, how many, and so on.

- Situations in which the PN may transfer the PN role to another nurse.

In the beginning it helped to be very transparent and tell staff: We don't know what we're doing, and you need to help us figure out what we're doing. When we started this, staff thought if you were on a council you were telling them what to do. But when we promoted transparency—"We're all in it together; please help us"—the staff took our cause to heart. Everyone did their part in bringing suggestions back to the drawing board. Even if everyone wasn't in agreement, they still tried just about everything. That was a huge success.

—*Kirsten Roblee, BSN, RN, OCN*
Primary Nurse at OSUCCC—James

Educating Colleagues

Throughout your planning process, continue to expand the UPC's and staff's knowledge of Primary Nursing through staff meetings, bulletin boards, posters, email updates, articles, and presentations. Identify educational needs on specific topics, such as therapeutic relationships, effective communication, leadership, and healthy interpersonal relationships. Link your plan with national standards and the Nurse Practice Act to ensure that the professional standards are integrated into the plans for care delivery. Managers and educators are ready to help with education; ask them for the help you need.

Refining Outcome Measures

Another one of the UPC's duties is to gather baseline data on unit-specific measures, particularly questions on the patient satisfaction survey that reflect communication and how the patient perceives the care from nurses. This baseline data will be necessary in assessing the impact of your implementation and in guiding continuous performance improvement. Measure what is meaningful, share your findings widely, and make the needed changes based on the results.

UPCs will be expected to identify several unit-based outcome indicators that will best help your department measure the success of your plan. Assistance in measurement is likely available from your leadership team and the quality experts in your organization. Here are some ideas:

- Consider choosing two or three specific questions from your organization's patient satisfaction survey that are most likely to be impacted by your implementation of Primary Nursing.

- Use patient comment cards or post-visit phone calls to gather information about how the patient and family experienced Primary Nursing in your department.

- At discharge, ask the patient or family to identify the name of their Primary Nurse and to describe the relationship. (You'll find an excellent example in Appendix D.)

- Choose measures to evaluate the impact of your plan in improving collegial relationships and interdisciplinary collaboration. (For an example, see the Commitment to My Co-worker Healthy Team Assessment Survey [Koloroutis, 2004] in Appendix E.)

- Include key patient clinical outcomes specific to your department. A few examples of outcome measures are:

  » Fewer visits or readmissions

  » Reduced infections or falls

  » Ownership by patients for following their plan of care

  » Medication accuracy

  » Achieving core measures

Progress Checks: Inspiring Ownership and Sharing Ideas

A proven practice to support successful planning is for all the UPCs to meet with the Primary Nursing coordinating committee and the Primary Nursing implementation leader, two or three times during the planning phase. The purpose of these progress checks is to provide expert objective review, encouragement, and guidance. In addition, councils can hear one another's ideas and receive just-in-time education for the next steps.

Objectives of Progress Checks

- Communicate accomplishments to date and share creative ideas.

- Affirm and celebrate learning and accomplishments.

- Identify support needed from others in the organization.

- Receive education and ideas to make implementation plans even more successful.

- Prepare for the official presentation of plans to implement Primary Nursing.

It's important to share ideas with other units. In the beginning we were very guarded about sharing our ideas, but that has changed over time. We've learned so much from each other. Sharing ideas about Primary Nursing has brought units together; people are communicating like they never have before. That whole notion of "mine" needs to go out the window.

—*Dena Uscio, BBA, RN, OCN*
Primary Nurse at OSUCCC—James

Two or three progress checks during the planning period (about every six to eight weeks) tend to reinspire councils and serve as accountability checkpoints. These meetings should be positive, energizing, and educational in nature. They make a huge difference in instilling confidence and creativity, overcoming barriers, and assuring that each department is on track. Progress check meetings should be facilitated by a dynamic leader at any level who has a clear vision of and expertise in Primary Nursing.

Presenting Your Plan

Once the principles and questions in Appendix C have been discussed and your unit-specific plan is completed, the day of formal implementation is just ahead. It's time for the UPC to present their plan to key leaders and to the Primary Nursing coordinating committee.

Now is the time to pause and review your work and the factors critical to your success so far. You will have completed discussion of the questions in Appendix C in preparation for your presentation.

The Presentation Process

Before implementation, you will share your unit-specific plans in a formal presentation to the Primary Nursing coordinating committee, other UPCs, and other organizational leaders. You will have kept the council, your manager, and your colleagues informed of your progress. Now is the time to pause and share all of your action plans. The purpose of the pause is to reflect and make sure the plans are consistent with the overarching mission and values of the organization and the principles of Primary Nursing. Managers will also present their plans to support and sustain implementation.

- Presentations will be scheduled for each unit's UPC and manager to share their unique plan for implementing and sustaining Primary Nursing.

- All UPCs should attend all presentations so that they can learn from one another.

- Presentations should adhere to the following suggested outline but should be creative in style. PowerPoint slides and handouts are recommended.

The Presentation Outline

- Make introductions of all UPC members, including names and roles.

- Report your success in engaging all of your peers in creating the plan. What methods of communication worked well?

- Respectfully and appreciatively describe the care delivery system used before Primary Nursing. (Be careful not to disparage the prior system because those who designed and/or championed it may be present.)

- Share your vision for Primary Nursing. Focus on how it supports your organization's nursing philosophy and goals.

- Share detailed plans, organized around each element of the care delivery system. While much of your plan will be unique to your department, the following components of the plan are essential to include:

  » Primary Nursing responsibilities.

  » Criteria for assigning Primary Nurses to new patients.

- » Timing for assigning Primary Nurses to new patients.

- » Introduction of Primary Nursing to patients and families.

- » System for communicating who is the Primary Nurse for each patient.

- » How the Primary Nurse will learn about the patient as a person.

- » How patients will be involved in the plan of care and all decisions.

- » Documentation, communication, and handoffs.

- Share how you and your manager will collaborate to educate about and spread Primary Nursing.

- Share your plan for outcome measurement.

- Offer closing thoughts and reflections.

Preparation for Implementation: Final Polishing

Each UPC should make any adjustments to their plan recommended by others so that the unit-specific plan is consistent with the organization design prior to implementation. Furthermore, members may have heard an idea from other UPCs during the presentations that they would like to incorporate into their plan. The plan should be in writing so that it can be communicated to all staff and used for the orientation of new staff and as a guide for continuous improvement.

> People just need to know that Primary Nursing is an ever changing thing. You don't just do it. We were "Wave 1" of Primary Nursing and we are still changing our Primary Nursing model.
>
> —*Kirsten Roblee, BSN, RN, OCN*
> *Primary Nurse at OSUCCC—James*

Once again, UPC members use the communication network to:

- Acknowledge everyone's contributions.

- Inform all team members about final plans.

- Answer any questions.

- Articulate expectations for the full implementation of the plan.

"Go Live" Day

Implementation begins on a "Go Live" day selected by the UPC in conjunction with the manager. On that day, the plans developed by the UPC are fully implemented in the department.

This is a day to do the following:

- Put into place all the action plans for each of the elements of the Primary Nursing care delivery system.

- Begin assigning each patient to a Primary Nurse.

- Update or eliminate practices that are no longer in keeping with the implementation plan.

- Engage all colleagues in the department in a celebration: nurses, physicians, clinical professionals, and support staff.

The UPC's Role in Sustaining Primary Nursing

The UPC will continue to meet regularly after implementation to evaluate, model, and fully integrate the Primary Nursing care delivery system. During implementation, staff members may need frequent reminders and reinforcement of the new practices. Often they need to unlearn old behaviors and begin new behaviors that may feel uncomfortable at first. They will need help and encouragement from both the manager and UPC members.

> The discomfort in Primary Nursing, when it's just getting started ... the awkwardness in it is a good thing because it means you're getting over or through all of the reasons that have kept you from doing patient-centered care in the first place. In general, the discomfort and challenges and difficulties are not signs of failure, but signs of success.
>
> —*Nicole Vance*, BSN, RN
> *Primary Nurse at UC Davis Medical Center*

The UPC's Role in Initiating Case Presentations

One extremely helpful sustainment activity is case presentations. Although the manager is involved in scheduling these events and Primary Nurses are responsible for preparing and presenting them, members of the UPC should take the lead in modeling the first round of case presentations, thereby setting the stage for all Primary Nurses to participate in subsequent presentations.

Case Presentations to Strengthen Primary Nursing and Professional Practice

Format. Case presentations last ten to fifteen minutes and are presented by the Primary Nurse. They involve recently discharged patients, never current patients. An educational focus explores what can be learned from the care decisions made by the Primary Nurse. Case presentations can be given as individual events at staff meetings or as part of continuing education events with multiple case presentations.

Case presentations summarize these points:

1. Patient's social situation (patient as a person).

2. Patient's medical history (brief).

3. Patient problems/needs which the Primary Nurse identified.

4. What the Primary Nurse did that worked and anything that did not work.

5. How collaboration with others enhanced the care of the patient.

6. Lessons learned.

A sample case presentation can be found in Appendix F.

Implementation Tips

Once the implementation has been underway for a reasonable amount of time (typically two to four months), the UPC performs a comprehensive review, using I_2E_2, of the principles and action steps that have been put into practice.

The UPC should resist the urge to make subsequent adaptations too quickly. New systems require time to settle in and become comfortable, and it may be discovered that a plan is sound, even if initial adherence to it is weak. Continue using your communication network for feedback before making any changes. Some decisions will work well. Others may need to be revisited and revised during continuous improvement. Primary Nursing will continue to evolve over time as the UPC and staff members review and reflect on the impact of Primary Nursing on patients and staff. Continuous learning, development, and thoughtful refinement—not perfection—are the goals. (See Figure 4.3.)

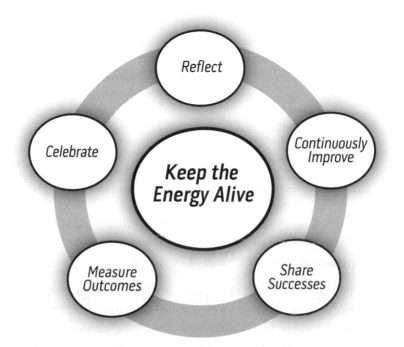

Figure 4.3: Keys to Deepening and Sustaining Primary Nursing

Summary of Key Points

- Two groups will play a significant role in the design and implementation of Primary Nursing in each department. The unit practice council (UPC) guides the design of how care will be delivered in an individual department, and the coordinating committee provides oversight at the organizational or system level to ensure that the principles of Primary Nursing provide the core of practice.

- UPC members must be educated about:
  - » council responsibilities and scope
  - » levels of authority

> » leadership roles

> » leading an effective meeting

> » communicating with all their peers

> » taking minutes

> » leading change

> » decision-making methods

> » systems of accountability (Wessel, 2012)

- The Primary Nursing coordinating committee includes people who have vast experience with and/or show unwavering advocacy for Primary Nursing.

- A comprehensive list of questions helps teams understand how the following elements will be expressed in practice: (1) responsibility for relationship and decision making, (2) work allocation and patient assignments, (3) communication with the health care team, and (4) management and leadership philosophy.

- Colleagues must be provided with education on therapeutic relationships, effective communication, leadership, and healthy interpersonal relationships.

- Determine outcomes that will be measured in order to show the impact of Primary Nursing in your department.

- Two or three progress checks during the planning period (about every six to eight weeks) reinspire councils and serve as accountability checkpoints.

- After your implementation plan is complete, you will pause to reflect and make sure the plans are consistent with the overarching mission and values of the organization and the principles of Primary Nursing.

- UPCs will continue to meet regularly after implementation has begun in order to evaluate, model, and fully integrate the Primary Nursing care delivery system.

- Case presentations are used to strengthen Primary Nursing and professional practice by providing opportunities for learning, reflection, and discussion about the care of recently discharged patients.

Questions for Reflection

- Think about or discuss how greater continuity of care could result in a decreased workload for caregivers.

- Who are the people in your organization who are already enthusiastic advocates of Primary Nursing? How might they be able to facilitate a sense of enthusiasm for Primary Nursing in others?

- What are the benefits of having the department-specific plan for Primary Nursing designed by the people who will use the system? Why is customization for each unit so important?

- If you are a Primary Nurse (or about to be one), what are your thoughts about having more autonomy in decision making? What are you excited about? What are your concerns?

- Think about or discuss what questions from your organization's patient satisfaction survey would most likely be impacted by your implementation of Primary Nursing.

- How do you feel about the fact that Primary Nursing requires continual reenvisioning by the unit practice council? Identify people in your department or organization who seem particularly adept at the improvement of systems and processes.

When the infrastructure worked and Primary Nurses got their patients, no complaints. When Primary Nurses didn't get their patients, lots of complaints.

KIRSTEN ROBLEE, BSN, RN, OCN
PRIMARY NURSE AT OSUCCC—JAMES

Chapter 5

Primary Nursing Implementation: The Manager's Role

Three factors help to ensure the successful implementation of Primary Nursing:

1. Leadership is organized around decentralized decision making.

2. Members of management have a commitment toward Primary Nursing to "support without pressure" and a nonpunitive attitude toward human error.

3. Appropriate council structures and functions are established that include leadership at all levels.

It is important to understand the role and responsibilities of the first-line manager (whatever his or her title is) in a culture of decentralized decision making. First-line managers must be skilled in both the leadership and management aspects of their roles. In the broadest sense, the staff's role is to manage the patients, and the manager's role is to lead the staff. How well first-line managers perform their role can make or break a department and its success in practicing Primary Nursing. While it is true that a unit *can* implement Primary Nursing without the support of the organization, it is also true that a unit *cannot* implement Primary Nursing without the support of its manager.

> *A unit cannot implement Primary Nursing without the support of its manager.*

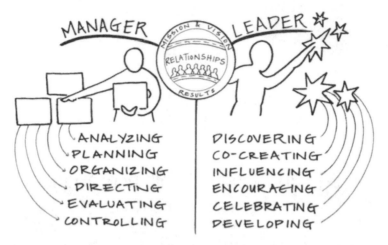

Figure 5.1: Manager Roles vs. Leader Roles

See Figure 5.1. You will notice that relationships are at the center of this image. Having healthy interpersonal relationships and being a role model for caring are the foundations of a manager's success.

First-line management is perhaps the most difficult role in health care. The span of control and the complexity of relationships, not to mention the fast pace of change, can be daunting. A manager's success is greatly helped by understanding and using decentralized decision making—that is, having a successful unit-level shared governance council to take on decisions about patient care and systems. Success is also enhanced by a clearly articulated shared vision that is grounded in professional practice standards and ethics.

Decentralized Decision Making

In shared governance, also called shared decision making or decentralized decision making, the manager trusts first-line staff to make decisions about how Primary Nursing should be implemented in their departments. The manager assists in establishing a unit-based council structure and serves as an advisor or guide, helping the council to be successful. This is quite different from participatory leadership.

*In a decentralized shared decision-making culture,
decisions are made at the level of action by people in the best
position to judge their outcomes.*

GEN GUANCI, MEd, RN-BC, CCRN-K

Figure 5.2 distinguishes participatory leadership from shared governance. Take particular note of the differences in the manager's role in each structure. The table, which is taken from Gen Guanci's book, *Feel the Pull*, has been adapted to address the particular concerns of managers in units implementing Primary Nursing.

	Participatory Leadership	Shared Governance
Goals	Managers request input from staff; use of input is optional.	Staff members are given responsibility and authority for decisions within their circle of influence.
Use of Input	Manager is not required to use staff input.	Manager and staff activities are interdependent.
How Decisions Are Made	Final decision lies with manager and/or management team.	Managers clearly articulate the guidelines for the decision. Staff decisions are honored.
Status of Leader	Hierarchical leadership	Transformational leader
Where Decisions Are Made	Centralized decision making	Decentralized decision making

Figure 5.2: Guanci's Participatory Leadership vs. Shared Governance Analysis
Source: Adapted from: Guanci, G. (2007). *Feel the pull: Creating a culture of nursing excellence.* Minneapolis, MN: Creative Health Care Management, p. 64.

The implementation of Primary Nursing is a perfect arena for decentralized decision making. The decision to choose this nursing care delivery system is often made by top nurse executives in collaboration with staff. How to make it come to life must be planned by direct caregivers—in this case, through the work of a unit practice council (UPC). The UPC plans the details of Primary Nursing, carefully seeking input from all members of the staff using a comprehensive communication network.

Attitudes of Members of the Management Team

Years of experience in implementing this care delivery system have taught us that implementation will be greatly facilitated when management team members start out with the belief that nurses want to take good care of their patients. Trusting first-line caregivers to make decisions about how Primary Nursing will work demonstrates this positive belief. This means that the manager leads and supports the implementation process by conveying respect for the team and guiding them without exerting managerial pressure.

A second contributor to successful implementation is that managers demonstrate a nonpunitive attitude toward human error. Mistakes in clinical judgment are inherent in professional practice because decisions must often be made before there is time to acquire all of the relevant data and information. Managers must use mistakes in clinical judgment as opportunities for reflection and learning. This is different from procedural mistakes, which may indicate the need for education or system improvements.

> Managers must use mistakes in clinical judgment as opportunities for reflection and learning.

Amy Edmundson, in her book *Teaming: How Organizations Learn, Innovate, and Compete in the Knowledge Economy* (2012), describes mistakes (failure) as essential for innovation and learning. She writes that it is important for managers to understand the context-specific responses to failures. She defines three types of failures: (1) preventable (caused by a lack of skill, not following procedure, a lack of support), (2) complex, as a result of system breakdowns that may not be recognized in time for preventive actions (i.e., sentinel events that require deconstruction and analysis), and (3) intelligent mistakes or unsuccessful trials that occur as part of thoughtful design and implementations that provide opportunity for learning and refinement (pp. 164–165). The manager and the team need to understand the importance of intelligent mistakes as part of innovation and create an environment that is supportive of taking appropriate risks. One of the biggest impediments to a successful implementation can be the fear that professional nurses experience when their name goes on a whiteboard or chart as the person who has accepted responsibility for managing the care of the patient. Healthy reflection, openly sharing lessons, and support from managers to do so will help staff members be courageous decision makers.

Responsibilities of Managers

To be effective, empowered leaders, managers must have the skills to perform these core competencies (see Figure 5.3). In some situations, these responsibilities may be delegated to others with appropriate oversight.

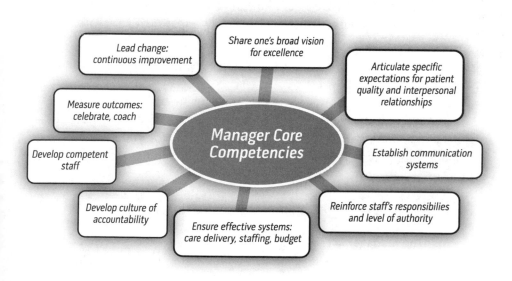

Figure 5.3: Manager Responsibilities

The Manager's Responsibilities for Primary Nursing

We encourage you to present your plan for leading and sustaining Primary Nursing only after your unit practice council presents its plan for implementation. The foundation for your plan is a set of principles for managing a department with a Primary Nursing care delivery system. These principles are a guide for your decisions about how you will carry out your responsibilities in managing this transition and sustaining it.

A unique responsibility of nurse managers is that of clinical leadership. If you are a manager, you and only you are charged with determining how nursing care is delivered to the patients in your department and for continuously improving that care. A Primary Nursing care delivery system provides a means to achieve highly professional ethical and personalized care.

Our manager is pretty adamant now, that if you choose to work here, you choose to be family-centered and use Primary Nursing, and if that doesn't work for you—(she's very diplomatic about it, but...)—you have an option to look for another job. For our unit, it's run that way, so even with the nurses who have a hard time, it comes back to the fact that it's not about the nurse; it's about the family, and it's patient-centered.

—*Heidi Nolen, BSN, RN*
Primary Nurse at UC Davis Medical Center

Successful implementation of Primary Nursing requires specific decisions and actions by managers. This chapter will guide you through those responsibilities and give you tools to determine a plan for your role in this process.

Principles of Management Related to Primary Nursing

1. The manager actively and visibly supports shared governance and the success of the unit practice council in implementing Primary Nursing.

2. The manager articulates expectations for Primary Nursing based on the plan developed by the UPC. The manager oversees full implementation, taking action to measure what matters, celebrate successes, and coach the team and individual members of the staff as needed.

3. The manager promotes professional practice and reinforces the responsibilities of Primary Nurses for:

   » Establishing a therapeutic relationship and personalized care.

   » Developing a plan of care in partnership with the patient.

   » Collaborating with individuals in other professional disciplines.

4. The manager establishes clear expectations for a healthy work environment that includes teamwork, mutual respect, and open, honest communication.

5. The manager measures the effectiveness of Primary Nursing on patient safety, the patient experience, and the quality of care. Outcomes are used as a source of reinforcement and inspiration.

6. The manager provides and supports learning opportunities to deepen the knowledge of Primary Nursing. Staff members are encouraged to continuously improve their practice and reflect on successes and failures as opportunities to learn.

The following pages contain a small sampling of questions, the answers to which will become the basis of the manager's action plan for supporting implementation of Primary Nursing. A full list of questions can be found in Appendix G. Note that the unit practice council, not the manager, has the responsibility for determining the action plan for how Primary Nursing will work day to day.

Questions for Reflection to Develop Manager Action Plan

Principle 1

The manager actively and visibly supports shared governance and the success of the unit practice council in implementing Primary Nursing.

Questions
How will I enable meetings of the UPC, balancing the needs of patients and the council?   How will I find out what the council needs from me in order to be successful?   How will I follow up on issues or barriers identified by the UPC that are beyond their scope and get them solved?   See Appendix G for the full list of questions.

Principle 2

The manager articulates expectations for Primary Nursing based on the plan developed by the UPC. The manager oversees full implementation, taking action to measure what matters, celebrate successes, and coach staff as needed.

Questions
What are all of my opportunities to communicate in words and actions my expectations that Primary Nursing will be fully embraced for all patients?   In what ways can I reinforce the spread of Primary Nursing and learn about the success of nurses in carrying out this new role?   How can I help and encourage those who are reluctant to adopt this role?   See Appendix G for the full list of questions.

Principle 3

The manager promotes professional practice and reinforces the responsibilities of Primary Nurses for:

1. Establishing a therapeutic relationship and personalized patient care.

2. Developing a plan of care in partnership with the patient.

3. Collaborating with individuals in other disciplines.

Questions
How can I assess individual nurses' success in developing a therapeutic and trusting relationship with patients and families? How can I observe and reinforce transdisciplinary and interdepartmental communication and collaboration? See Appendix G for the full list of questions.

Principle 4

The manager establishes clear expectations for a healthy work environment that includes teamwork, mutual respect, and open, honest communication.

Questions
Has the UPC translated the organization's values and beliefs about interpersonal relationships into specific behavioral expectations? How can I convey my expectations that staff will be responsible for managing their interpersonal relationships consistent with our articulated values and beliefs? What process will I use to assess and recognize those who are following our behavioral expectations? What process will I use when individuals have a pattern of consistently not following our agreed-upon behaviors? See Appendix G for the full list of questions.

There are some staff members who feel that complex care coordination patients shouldn't have a Primary Nurse who only works nights. They feel that the bulk of the problems that happen, happen on the day shift. That's something that my manager has decided to never get in the middle of—to never say who can or can't be a Primary Nurse.

—*Nicole Vance,* BSN, RN
Primary Nurse at UC Davis Medical Center

Principle 5

The manager measures the effectiveness of Primary Nursing on patient safety, the patient experience, and the quality of care. Outcomes are used as a source of reinforcement and inspiration.

Questions
What measures are most important in assessing whether each patient and/or family experiences the impact of the Primary Nurse relationship? How will I participate in collecting these outcomes? How will I use outcome data to inspire staff and others? What will I do if outcomes do not show improvement? See Appendix G for the full list of questions.

Principle 6

The manager provides and supports learning opportunities to deepen knowledge of Primary Nursing. Staff members are encouraged to continuously improve their practice and reflect on successes and failures as opportunities for learning.

Questions
In what ways will I support and help educate the entire team in practicing Primary Nursing? In what ways can we deepen our insights about the primary relationship and model reflective practice? See Appendix G for the full list of questions.

If you have successfully answered the questions in Appendix G and developed a plan, you are well on your way to fulfilling your leadership responsibilities for ensuring a successful implementation. We recommend collaborating with other managers as they develop their plans, so that you can share ideas with one another before you present your final plan and put it into action.

Refining Outcome Measures

In collaboration with your UPC, baseline data should be gathered on the unit-specific measures you have identified. This baseline data is necessary to assess the impact of your plan and to guide the continuous performance improvement process. Measure what is meaningful, share results widely, and make needed changes based on the results.

You and your council will be expected to identify several unit-based outcome indicators that will best help you measure the success of your plan. Support is available from your Primary Nursing coordinating committee and/or the quality experts in your organization. Here are some ideas:

- Choose two or three specific questions from your organization's patient satisfaction survey that you believe are most likely to be impacted by your plan.

- Measure the impact of Primary Nursing by asking the patient or family at discharge to identify the name of the Primary Nurse and to describe the relationship.

- Choose measures to evaluate the impact of your plan in improving collegial relationships and interdisciplinary collaboration.

- Consider current clinical outcomes and how they will improve with Primary Nursing and more personal, consistent relationships.

> Recently I changed the audit a little, and now we ask, "Has the Primary Nurse decreased your anxiety during treatment?" That way we have a nurse-sensitive indicator we're tracking. Ever since we've added that question, 100% of the patients indicated that their Primary Nurse has helped to reduce their anxiety.
>
> —*Kathleen Fowler, BSN, RN*
> *Primary Nurse at OSUCCC—James*

Progress Check Meetings

Evidence of progress by the UPC is shared during meetings with your Primary Nursing coordinating committee two or three times during the planning phase. The purpose of these meetings is to provide objective feedback, encouragement, and guidance. Managers should attend these meetings with their UPC and be prepared to share their progress in developing the management plan for supporting Primary Nursing. Your presence at progress checks and communication of your plan demonstrate your support and commitment to Primary Nursing and the work of the UPCs.

Presenting Your Management Plan

Before implementation, a time should be scheduled to pause and share your unit-specific plans in a formal presentation to the Primary Nursing coordinating committee, other UPCs, and other organizational leaders. The purpose of the pause is to reflect and make sure the plans are consistent with the overarching mission and values of the organization and the management principles of Primary Nursing. UPC members will also present their plans for implementation.

During your presentation:

- Share the successes to be celebrated.

- Describe how you will carry out the management principles related to Primary Nursing.

- Note any related issues and obstacles you have identified.

- Discuss the support and assistance needed for a successful implementation.

Keep in mind that you may hear an idea from another manager during the presentations that you would like to incorporate into your plan. Make any adjustments recommended by others that will enhance your plan.

Case Presentation: Developing Nurses' Skill and Confidence in Being a Primary Nurse

Case presentations are a proven strategy for deepening Primary Nursing practice and encouraging critical thinking and reflection. Case presentations should be held regularly after implementation of Primary Nursing to share experiences, develop newer staff members, and encourage self-reflection. They also reinforce the independent realm of nursing practice and professional accountability. The nurse manager is responsible for collaborating with the UPC to schedule case presentations.

Case presentations were discussed in more depth in Chapter 4, and an example of a case presentation can be found in Appendix F.

Empowering Your Team is the Key to Your Success

Hopefully this chapter has helped you reflect on how to practice decentralized decision making to achieve Primary Nursing. You have enabled your UPC to decide the details of implementation. You have also developed a thoughtful plan about how you can ensure their success.

Now your ultimate leadership role will be to set clear and inspiring expectations for Primary Nursing in your department, to actively support decisions made by your UPC about the details, and to support complete implementation by coaching staff members as they learn the Primary Nurse role. You will now have the pleasure of seeing staff members grow as leaders and professional practitioners.

> I really feel that we have wonderful management. They supported our UPC and whatever we initiated. They trusted that we know the work. They helped us do retreats and helped the UPC to get off-unit time. That kind of support from management really helps to get things off the ground.
>
> *—Jane Czekajewski, BSN, RN, CNOR*
> *Primary Nurse at OSUCCC—James*

Summary of Key Points

- In a culture of shared governance/decentralized decision making, first-line managers must be skilled in both the leadership and management aspects of their roles.

- The manager actively and visibly supports shared governance and the success of the unit practice council in implementing Primary Nursing.

- The manager articulates expectations for Primary Nursing based on the plan developed by the UPC. The manager oversees full implementation, taking action to measure what matters, celebrate successes, and coach staff as needed.

- The manager promotes professional practice and reinforces the responsibilities of Primary Nurses for establishing a therapeutic relationship and personalized patient care, developing a plan of care in partnership with the patient/family, and collaborating with individuals in other professional disciplines.

- The manager measures the effectiveness of Primary Nursing with regard to patient safety, the patient experience, and the quality of care. Outcomes are used as a source of reinforcement and inspiration.

- The manager provides and supports learning opportunities to deepen knowledge of Primary Nursing. Staff members are encouraged to continuously improve their practice and reflect on successes and failures as opportunities for learning.

Questions for Reflection

- Compare and contrast leadership and management. Why is having skills in both of them so important for managers of departments implementing Primary Nursing?

- Why is it important for managers to develop their own plans for leading and sustaining Primary Nursing? How will that differ from the work of the unit practice council?

- What can managers do to proactively inspire their staff members to create and sustain Primary Nursing in their departments?

If something doesn't work, and you gave it a fair chance,
try something else.

JANE CZEKAJEWSKI, BSN, RN, CNOR
PRIMARY NURSE AT OSUCCC—JAMES

Chapter 6

How Ancillary Professionals and Service Staff Are Adapting Primary Nursing Principles in Their Departments

The impact of patients having a primary caregiver is nearly as strong for other clinical professionals as it is for nurses. When patients know which therapist, which physician, or which social worker is coordinating their care, the visible interconnection of the team creates a safe haven for the patient and family, increasing their sense of trust and emotional safety (Koloroutis & Trout, 2012).

In addition, we have observed that care is safer, there is less duplication of efforts, and patients have better outcomes when there is a primary caregiver from each discipline. Because of the continuity of each relationship over time, the primary caregiver develops a deeper and more accurate understanding of the patient and family. For example, when a primary respiratory therapist works with a patient who has asthma or COPD, that therapist gains clinical insight not merely about "people with asthma or COPD" but about how this specific patient functions with these specific conditions. Being intimately familiar with what is normal for this specific patient, the primary caregiver may recognize much sooner the early signs of respiratory difficulty and know which measures are most effective in heading off a full-scale asthma attack or pneumonia for this person. The very same principles have made the Patient-Centered Medical Home model so effective in ambulatory settings.

We have worked with people from diverse clinical disciplines who have developed systems for primary or lead caregivers. In our work in the field, we have seen staff councils do marvelous work in pharmacy, psychology, counseling, social service, audiology, physical and occupational therapy, nutrition, phlebotomy, imaging technology, radiation oncology, and respiratory care in order to ensure that patients experience greater continuity within their care teams. The outcomes for both patients and the professionals serving in this role have been significant. Some have used the term "primary," others call it "lead," and still others use the term "designated liaison." The nomenclature is not important; rather, what is important is that the designation encourages the person to take responsibility for (1) individual ownership for knowing the patient, (2) knowing what is important to the patient, (3) overall coordination of care for each discipline, and (4) collaboration across disciplines for the benefit of the patient.

Exemplars from Clinical Services

Pharmacy: Primary Pharmacists

Councils of staff pharmacists and pharmacy techs in many hospitals have created innovative ways of enhancing their roles through the creation of a Primary Pharmacist role. Since this happens within existing staffing and budget, a realistic way to approach it is by having a Primary Pharmacist for protocol patients (patients who are on medication protocols that require education by a pharmacist, such as those going on Coumadin).

To share a wonderful example, a medical center piloted the Primary Pharmacist role by assigning a clinical pharmacist to a large medical surgical unit. The program was later expanded to other units because it was such a resounding success. There was no physical space for satellite pharmacies, so Primary Pharmacists split their time between the main pharmacy and the nursing unit; pharmacy software was installed in a computer on the nursing unit. The Primary Pharmacist's time was spent in a very innovative way:

FIRST HALF OF MORNING

Primary Pharmacist is on the nursing unit, meeting new patients and explaining his or her role as Primary Pharmacist, communicating directly with physicians and nurses about orders, writing pharmacy goals for each patient on the interdisciplinary form, and participating in interdisciplinary rounds.

SECOND HALF OF MORNING

Primary Pharmacist returns to pharmacy to process orders since this is the heavy workload time for pharmacy.

AFTERNOON

Primary Pharmacist checks with unit secretary to learn which patients are being discharged. Reviews discharge medication orders, catching any problems and helping reconcile medications before the patient leaves. Primary Pharmacist visits and meets new patients, and completes any needed patient education.

Two immediate results of the pilot were improved relationships between pharmacy and nursing and reports of numerous corrections of potential issues with discharge medication orders before the patient left. It is worth noting that some of the incorrect medication orders involved duplication of medications patients were already getting through their Primary Physicians. The new orders were sometimes in the same family of drugs and would have caused a significant overdose had they not been caught.

Social Service: Lead Social Worker

A social work department in a VA medical center had a strong existing system of permanently assigning its social workers to the same patients, as most health care organizations do. They decided to take the benefits of having a relationship with a primary social worker to a much deeper level with a group of their most complex patients.

Administration had identified a small group of veterans who were very heavy users of VA services, some of them coming into the ED almost weekly. Their problems were both psychosocial and physical. The staff council of social workers created a new process for one Lead Social Worker to follow a small group of veterans using a strengths-based Veteran Change Model. The program was designed, individual patients were contacted and invited, and the Lead Social Worker worked with them both individually and in group sessions. The Lead Social Worker facilitated the creation of individual goals and provided mentoring based on the personalized health goals of each veteran. Participating veterans were surveyed at the beginning, midpoint, and end of the process; additional outcomes measured included the number of hospital admissions and emergency department visits.

At the completion of the program, over 50% of the participants had fewer hospital admissions and ED visits. They were developing more skills along with the resilience necessary to take ownership of their health. The program outcomes were presented at a professional conference, and approval was obtained to replicate the process with another group of veterans with highly complex needs.

Respiratory Therapy: Lead Therapist

Respiratory therapy departments often schedule their staff members to rotate to different departments each day, enabling them to maintain their clinical skills in any specialty. Although this provides a benefit for the respiratory therapist, it means that patients see a different therapist every day. Having worked with numerous respiratory departments, we have seen the positive impact of redesigning schedules and implementing a Lead Therapist concept.

In one example, the respiratory staff council changed their assignments so that they spent an average of five days in a row assigned to the same department before rotating. They developed a letter to accompany their introduction as the patient's Lead Therapist. The letter explained the role of Lead Therapist, and the therapists filled in their names so that their patients would know them. They emphasized patient education, using computerized educational materials in a way that had not been done before. These therapists found themselves accepting responsibility for managing their patients' respiratory needs in a much more comprehensive way. They also saw improved outcomes as patients were much better prepared for discharge.

Exemplars from Support Services

The fundamental benefit of having consistent relationships with someone we serve can also be realized in support services. It has been inspiring to see staff members voluntarily accept the responsibility for the quality of care or service to another department or to a patient. We will share two examples that have shown a major impact.

Sterile Processing Service: Designated Liaisons

In a sterile processing service (SPS) department, the staff council decided to create the role of Primary Liaison to a few departments that were heavy users of their services. They began with the surgery department because they were the largest "customer" of this service.

Surgery was asked to identify one key contact person from their staff to be the liaison they would work with. They began by having both managers and the two newly designated liaisons meet briefly to discuss the program and its goals. After this, the two liaisons regularly discussed problems, needs, and how to resolve them. Their result was improved availability of the right equipment, in good working order and ready to use. Time spent in fixing daily problems dropped dramatically. Trust between the two departments and willingness to learn from each other created vastly improved systems and fewer delays in surgery from incorrect or unavailable supplies and equipment. The program was expanded to other departments, with other SPS employees stepping up to be liaisons. A broader though less measurable impact of this initiative was that the pride and sense of meaning experienced by the SPS staff improved. They were located in the basement and had not felt valued or seen by other departments. This work helped them to see and ultimately own the difference they made in the safety of every patient and the ability of other departments to do their work.

Hospital Security: Designated Liaisons

In an inner city hospital police services department, the staff council decided to create an Adopt-A-Unit program in which officers would volunteer to be liaisons to specific nursing departments. They described their ideas as follows:

Adopt-A-Unit

- Recruit officers to be a liaison between a unit and police services in order to address ongoing issues and improve relationships.

- Designated Liaison officers will work to improve communication flow between the unit and police services.

- Post the Designated Liaison officer's information in the unit's break room.

- Designated Liaisons will educate staff on police roles.

  » Safety

  » Fourth Amendment (search and seizure)

  » Parking policy

  » Any questions regarding our services

Interestingly, the rise of primary or lead caregivers in services besides nursing has not typically come through mandates but rather from innovations proposed and designed by first-line staff members. When teams are empowered to restructure their work to provide the best possible experience for patients and their families, they often land on a primary or lead system on their own. When they are empowered to improve their own work, they put themselves in the shoes of the patient and family and are often eager to restructure their work to improve the patient experience.

Innovative ways to spread the principles of primary relationships can be applied to most departments, particularly if a council of first-line staff members is coached and encouraged along the way. Over time, organizational improvements can be seen in the patient experience, quality and safety indicators, overall employee engagement, and reduced turnover.

Summary of Key Points

- When patients have a primary caregiver and/or service provider from each discipline, care is safer, there is less duplication of efforts, and patients have better outcomes.

- Primary caregiver/service provider delivery systems have been successfully implemented for pharmacists, social workers, respiratory therapists, sterile processing and supply providers, and hospital security officers, to name only a few.

- Most primary caregiver/service provider delivery systems have not come through mandates from the organization. Most have been innovations proposed and designed by first-line staff members.

Questions for Reflection

- What ancillary and service areas in your organization might benefit from adopting a primary caregiver mindset and ways of delivering services?

As soon as the family trusts you, the whole dynamic changes. They feel a calmness with you, and you feel it with them, and you can just go directly to your job without having to explain as many things because you've already established the trust factor and the relationship is formed. If you can build the trust and the relationship, it just makes even the hardest days easier.

HEIDI NOLEN, BSN, RN
PRIMARY NURSE AT UC DAVIS MEDICAL CENTER

Chapter 7

Therapeutic Relationships:
The Essence of the Primary Nurse Role

In Primary Nursing, a therapeutic relationship is established between an RN and an individual patient and his or her family. Within this relationship, the nurse has the responsibility to identify the patient's unique health needs and to communicate and coordinate those needs with other members of the health care team (Koloroutis, 2004). While it is universally accepted that a therapeutic relationship with the patient and family is an essential aspect of Primary Nursing, there has been very little written about what a therapeutic relationship actually looks like and/or how to initiate it within time-constrained and rapid-paced health care settings (Zolnierek, 2014). To address this lack, nurse leader Mary Koloroutis and child and family psychologist Michael Trout studied how to form authentic, compassionate connections that enable the patient and family to trust their caregivers and partner with them for the best possible care.

A therapeutic relationship gets to the heart of what caregiving means because it is focused on what is most important to the patient and what will optimize healing. The purpose of the therapeutic relationship is threefold: (1) to help people cope, (2) to help patients and their families gain understanding and insight into the meaning of the illness experience in their lives, and (3) to help patients and their families take ownership (to the degree possible) for their own health and well-being. A therapeutic relationship can exist in even the briefest patient–clinician encounter, but when the care delivery system is Primary Nursing, this relationship is easier to establish because the care delivery system is actually designed to ensure that the nurse–patient relationship is given the time, space, and structure to flourish.

We know, however, that a therapeutic relationship doesn't happen automatically just because a clinician has the opportunity to create one. It happens when the clinician is mindful and intentional in connecting *therapeutically* and when the relationship is grounded in sound knowledge and skills that can be learned and mastered. This relationship does not depend on inherent capacities or personal characteristics of caregivers. It is not about being "nice"; it is about being therapeutically focused and thus depends on the self-awareness, commitment, and development of individual clinicians.

> A therapeutic relationship doesn't happen automatically just because a clinician has the opportunity to create one.

In their groundbreaking book, *See Me as a Person: Creating Therapeutic Relationships with Patients and Their Families*, Koloroutis and Trout describe four practices that enable clinicians to intentionally establish this therapeutic connection even in time-constrained circumstances. These practices will be introduced shortly, followed by an example of how they were applied in the care of a patient and her family by a Primary Nurse.

The Four Practices that Create Therapeutic Relationships

A therapeutic relationship is like no other. In this unique relationship, the clinician offers "care, touch, compassion, presence, and any other act or attitude that would foster healing, and expects nothing in return" (Koloroutis, 2004). In order to connect with another, clinicians must have the ability to be open and accepting of the people in their care, meeting them exactly where they are. The four therapeutic practices enable clinicians to become and remain open, accepting, and present regardless of the person and/or circumstances. The four therapeutic practices are: attuning, wondering, following, and holding. (See Figure 7.1.) These practices constitute a way of thinking, of being, and of interacting (Koloroutis & Trout, 2012).

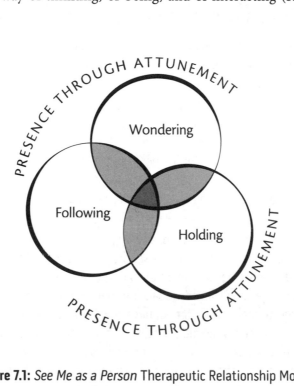

Figure 7.1: *See Me as a Person* Therapeutic Relationship Model

These intentional practices are not sequential, although the practice of attuning (noted in the model as "presence through attunement") is necessary for each of the other practices to occur. The three remaining practices will appear and reappear throughout the caregiving relationship, in any order and in every combination.

Attuning

Attuning to another person requires presence, which enables a level of connection, even if temporary, that leads the clinician to resonate with the patient and the patient (usually) to resonate with the clinician. This active attunement creates an environment that must exist in order for the next three practices to be effective. Without attunement from caregivers, the patient and family may feel thoroughly abandoned, no matter what else is going on around them. Mary Koloroutis elaborated on some of the intricacies of attuning in a keynote address:

> It is through consciously attuning to the person in our care that we convey the essential messages in nursing and medicine: I see you. I am interested in you. I give you my full attention. I am here. You are safe.
>
> We attune with a person when we move ourselves into a physical and mental position to be able to catch on to their state of mind. We attune with a person when we remember that what may be routine for us is definitely not routine for the person needing care—in fact it could be life altering. We attune with a person when we consciously suspend our own needs and agenda and focus on the needs of the other.
>
> Attunement is familiar to us. We experience attunement with another when we feel seen, heard, and respected. When we experience others giving us their full attention, we are likely to feel calmer and more connected. Science has documented the experience of co-regulation that occurs when any two individuals are well-attuned. A mother notices and attunes to the mental state of her baby. The baby notices and internally experiences the mental state of his mother, and then attunes to her. They are locked into each other. Their neurologies connect. In the process, the mother acquires the strange and powerful capacity to actually regulate the mood, movements, and affect of her baby.
>
> Our experience as patients, when we are suffering, fearful, perhaps momentarily regressed and vulnerable, may be remarkably like the experience of an infant—we too seek attunement, perhaps more than anything else—searching, wondering about our safety. We may be hyper-vigilant, and only after we perceive that the other really genuinely cares about our well-being are we able to relate and connect. When that happens, a therapeutic relationship can begin. (Koloroutis personal communication, December 12, 2014)

Wondering

Wondering requires a genuine sense of interest and curiosity about the other person. It takes the place of any assumptions, prior conclusions, or overdependence on checklists. Wondering requires us to seek to understand, to inquire, to listen, and to think about what might lie behind a person's words or body language. Examples of what wondering may sound like in action are:

- "What is your biggest concern today?"

- "What is most important to you right now?"

- "What has been your past experience with this?"

- "What worries you?"

In order to truly wonder, we must believe that the patient has something important to teach us and that both we and the patient benefit from our discovery of it. Wondering helps us avoid judging, jumping to premature conclusions and diagnoses, and labeling others. When we are aware of our own potential prejudices and judgments, we are more able to actively suspend them so as not to allow them to interfere with our therapeutic connection.

> *In order to truly wonder, we must believe that the patient has something important to teach us and that both we and the patient benefit from our discovery of it.*

Following

Following involves remembering, respecting, and acting on what we learn while listening to, observing, and interacting with our patients and families. Our care, our conversation, and our decisions are based on what the patient has shared and taught us—the patient leads and we follow. We are driven not by our own agenda but rather by the cues and insights we have learned from wondering and paying attention. Following may appear in our caring as we say things such as:

- "When you said _____, I wondered ..."

- "I noticed ..."

- "Tell me more about ..."

- "You seem [sad, excited, worried, ...]. Is that true?"

Following involves the active effort of listening deeply and staying curious about (and not interrupting) what we see and hear. Like wondering, following is easier when we believe that the patient has something important to teach us and that the quality of care is improved through our learning what matters to this person.

Holding

Holding is creating a safe haven for the people in our care. We protect them from harm, accept them as they are, and work to preserve their dignity. Holding may take the form of honoring their confidences and being a steady, nonjudgmental presence. When holding, we may find ourselves saying things such as:

- "Of course you feel that way …"

- "I will make sure this is taken care of."

- "I am here."

- "I will stay with you."

- "I am your Primary Nurse."

I explain to new patients that I'll be their Primary Nurse throughout infusion— that I may not have them each time, but if they have any desire to see me, I'll do my best to stop in. I'll look to see when they're here so I can stop in to see them and say "Hi." I let them know that I'll do follow-up, that I look at their chart and talk to the other nurses throughout the time so even if I don't see them every time, I will be aware of any changes in their plan.

—*Kathleen Fowler*, BSN, RN
Primary Nurse at OSUCCC—James

Holding results when we remember that every encounter with a patient has a beginning, middle, and end. Times of transitioning are points of vulnerability for patients, who need to know what to expect next.

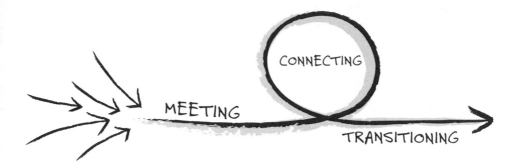

Figure 7.2: Three Phases of the Therapeutic Relationship

When transitions are not well attended to, anxiety is increased. The Primary Nurse anticipates and prepares patients and families for transitions in the care experience. Holding requires us to remember the sacred trust that the patient has given us and to live up to that trust as best we can, based on each person's unique needs (Koloroutis & Trout, 2012).

Primary Nursing and Therapeutic Boundaries

A Primary Nursing care delivery system provides the structure in which therapeutic relationships can most effectively be established and nurtured. It is notable that in our interviews with Primary Nurses, we discovered a wealth of wisdom about how to maintain healthy boundaries with patients and their families even when their circumstances are particularly challenging. When the connection is strong, healthy therapeutic boundaries can help protect a nurse from burnout while still forging a strong, authentic connection. Conventional wisdom and even simple logic may tell you that to protect yourself emotionally within a potentially heartbreaking situation, your best course of action is to disengage, but Nicole Vance, an RN and Primary Nurse at UC Davis Medical Center, has learned that there are emotionally safe ways to stay deeply connected to her primary patients and families:

I can honestly say that you *can* connect with patients no matter how tragically or how frequently you lose them, if you do it in a way that is for their benefit and not for your own emotional satisfaction as a nurse. If you can build a connection based on "What does this family need?" not "I like these guys; let's be friends," then you can still honor the professional relationship and maintain a healthy boundary that gives you enough room to take care of yourself and still work there.

In figure 7.3 below, adapted from the National Council of State Boards of Nursing, 2004, Koloroutis and Trout provide nurses and other caregivers with a helpful tool for reflection (2012, pp. 388–389).

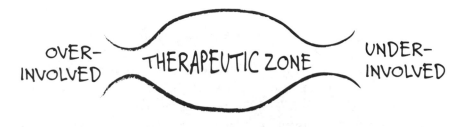

Figure 7.3: Therapeutic Zone

Again, Nicole Vance shares some thoughts that have helped her navigate the challenge of staying present and attuned in difficult circumstances without taking on the burdens of others:

It's a delicate balance between empathy with someone's struggles and ownership or responsibility for someone's struggles. If I'm not aware of that line on a regular basis, I'll cross it because I'm a nurse, and I want to help people feel better. It really comes down to putting yourself into their shoes, but not picking up their stuff.

The Story of a Therapeutic Relationship Created by a Primary Nurse, Told Through the Lenses of Attuning, Wondering, Following, and Holding

The following story brings to life the impact of a therapeutic relationship created by a nurse who has accepted responsibility for managing the care of her patient.

Patty was a 41-year-old attorney. Her Primary Nurse, Maya, was assigned to her when she came in for an exploratory surgery one year after her diagnosis of stomach cancer and a total gastrectomy. Two years previously, she and her husband had adopted twin girls who were now 4 years old. Patty and her husband were unwilling to discuss any end-of-life issues. They kept insisting there would be a miracle.

Attuning to this family meant meeting them right where they were and respecting their perspective. It would have been easy for Maya to see them as unrealistic in their hope for a miracle, but it would not have been helpful. In order for Maya to stay attuned to them, she needed to stay curious, open, and accepting.

When Maya or anyone on the team would approach the topic of end-of-life care, Patty absolutely refused to engage in those discussions and in fact threw her surgeon out of her room due to his persistence in approaching them about it. As Patty's Primary Nurse, Maya knew what mattered most to her. Maya respected Patty's and her family's right to move through this process in their own way and at their own rate, and she stepped in to advocate for them whenever she perceived that their wishes were not being heard and respected by others on the team.

The practice of **wondering** was key to helping Maya stay therapeutic. This family was making difficult decisions every day, and it would have closed down their relationship if Maya had judged Patty for being resistant, unrealistic, or "noncompliant," or if she moved in to fix, educate, or advise the family on their decisions. Instead, Maya connected with respect and openness. She continued to **wonder** as she related to this unique family working things out in their own way.

Several days into Patty's stay, as Maya asked Patty what was most important to her that day, Patty shared with Maya that they had planned to take the kids to Disneyland for their upcoming fifth birthday, and she asked Maya if she could help make that happen. That evening when her husband came, the three of them met, and with some degree of compromise, they figured out a way to make it happen. Patty wanted a picture of herself with the kids and Mickey Mouse so that they would always have this happy memory of her. They figured out what it would take, and they moved forward with a plan that included arranging for her husband to hook her up to a bag of fluid every night thru her implanted catheter, so that she wouldn't get too dehydrated. Some of the professionals involved in Patty's care (her surgeon, radiation oncologists, medical oncologists) thought this was a terrible idea, and some judged Maya especially harshly. But others, who had worked with Maya long enough to know that as a Primary Nurse she was always thoroughly tuned into her patients, trusted her decision. Patty's primary oncologist came to support the plan and wrote the necessary prescriptions and provided them with a contact in the area in case of an emergency.

All of this required adept **following** from Maya. She listened, respected, and acted upon what this patient and family told her was most important to them. The therapeutic benefits to the patient and family of Maya's following may be readily evident, but the benefits to Maya, her Primary Nurse, should not be overlooked. The more she listened, learned, and retained about Patty and her family, the more competent she was in their care. She understood the limits of Patty's current state better than anyone else, simply because, as her Primary Nurse, she had paid closer attention than anyone else had. Because she was so well informed, she confidently advocated for the family and empowered them as she took action to assure their safety in the event of an emergency.

Several days after their return, Patty landed in the hospital again. During this hospitalization, Maya talked with Patty and her husband about the importance of creating other memories related to what she would eventually leave behind for the children. With the trip accomplished, Patty was ready to consider this idea. While she remained hopeful for a miracle, the trip was clearly a turning point, giving her the peace she needed in order to move toward her inevitable death. She was able to write letters to each of the kids that they would open on significant events. Once this was done, Patty, her husband, and Maya were able to discuss other end-of-life issues such as where she wanted to die, whether she wanted hospice care in their home, whether she wanted the children there when she died, and how and when to tell the children that she was approaching death.

As a Primary Nurse, Maya experienced the distinct honor of **holding** this family in their most vulnerable hours. Because she stayed respectful of who they were, how they chose to live, and how Patty chose to die, she was able to be with them in a way that was supportive of them and ultimately healing for Patty. Maya served as a healer, guide, and advocate as she created a safe haven for Patty and her family to be together and work through important matters related to living and dying.

Maya's care of Patty and her family is an exquisite demonstration of a therapeutic relationship between a Primary Nurse and a patient and family. Clearly Maya's connection was informed by her expertise in oncology nursing and the dying process. Her professional knowledge enabled her to be mindful, present, and attuned as she guided and advocated for Patty's right to cope in her own way. Through all of her therapeutic interactions with Patty, Maya facilitated Patty's capacity to take ownership of herself and to actively mother her children through these final days of her life. The entire experience is one of Maya holding Patty and her loved ones in her care.

The Logical Combination of Primary Nursing and Therapeutic Relationships

The Primary Nursing care delivery system removes one of the biggest obstacles to the creation and development of therapeutic relationships—the lack of continuity of caregivers. It creates the ideal opportunity for therapeutic relationships to happen, and it is essential that we make the most of that opportunity. This chapter is a call to action for all those practicing Primary Nursing to learn, reflect on, practice, master, and then mentor the *See Me as a Person* practices for others. The purpose of Primary Nursing is to provide the best, most customized care for patients and families, and the therapeutic relationship practices provide the quickest route to fulfilling that purpose.

When an organization practices Primary Nursing and also educates those Primary Nurses in the four practices that create therapeutic relationships, the culture of that organization cannot help but be positively affected. All patients want caregivers who are competent technically. It is a minimum expectation. When asked what matters most, however, nearly all patients say they want to be seen, listened to, respected, and cared for with compassion. When we are patients, we expect that health care professionals—especially nurses and physicians—are knowledgeable in the human struggles inherent in needing care and that they will help us get through whatever we may be facing, whether physical or emotional. The implementation of Primary Nursing, combined with the *See Me as a Person* practices, guarantees healing culture in which patients and families truly are at the center of our care.

Summary of Key Points

- A therapeutic relationship does not depend on the inherent capacities or personal characteristics of caregivers. It is not about being "nice"; it is about being therapeutically focused and thus depends on the self-awareness, commitment, and development of individual clinicians.

- The four therapeutic practices explained in the book and workshop *See Me as a Person* are attuning, wondering, following, and holding. These practices constitute a way of thinking, of being, and of interacting.

- The active attunement of the caregiver must exist in order for the therapeutic practices of wondering, following, and holding to be effective.

- Without attunement from caregivers, the patient and family may feel abandoned, no matter what else is going on around them.

- The therapeutic practice of wondering helps us avoid judging, jumping to premature conclusions and diagnoses, and labeling others. When we are aware of our own potential prejudices and judgments, we are more able to actively suspend them so as not to allow them to interfere with our therapeutic connection.

- The therapeutic practice of following involves remembering, respecting, and acting on what we learn while listening to, observing, and interacting with our patients and families. It involves the active effort of listening deeply and staying curious about (and not interrupting) what we see and hear.

- The therapeutic practice of holding means creating a safe haven for the persons in our care. We protect them from harm, accept them as they are, and work to preserve their dignity. Holding may take the form of honoring their confidences and being a steady, nonjudgmental presence.

- Logic may tell you that in order to protect yourself emotionally in a potentially heartbreaking situation, your best course of action is to disengage, but if you can build a connection based on the patient's and family's needs rather than on forming a friendship, you can honor the professional relationship and maintain a healthy boundary.

- The implementation of Primary Nursing, combined with the *See Me as a Person* practices, guarantees a healing culture in which patients and families truly are at the center of our care.

Questions for Reflection

- In what ways are therapeutic relationships unlike any of our other relationships? Reflect on what privileged access we have to the lives of people who are vulnerable and suffering.

- Think of a therapeutic encounter in which you have used at least two of the therapeutic practices of attuning, wondering, following, and holding, even if you were not aware that you had done so.

- Explore the benefits of having strong therapeutic boundaries. How do strong boundaries actually make good therapeutic interactions possible?

- Reflect on the story of Patty and her family. Maya supported Patty in a belief that Maya knew was unrealistic. How was her support of such a thing therapeutic?

- Think about or discuss the ways in which a Primary Nursing care delivery system and the consistent use of the four therapeutic practices are a natural fit.

Part III:

Best Practices and Sustainment Strategies

We had a parent who would lay into whoever walked through the door. The verbal abuse was constant, so we kept a close eye on the Primary Nurse. We'd gauge how she was doing during the day, we'd run interference for her, we'd go into the room and do things for her. And when the child passed, we all went to the memorial. This method of taking care of each other has been largely informal and peer driven.

NICOLE VANCE, BSN, RN
PRIMARY NURSE AT UC DAVIS MEDICAL CENTER

Chapter 8

What's Working in the Real World: Best Practices from Successful Primary Nurses

It must be emphasized that the same practice that works beautifully in one unit or department may not work in every setting. Primary Nursing details must be tailored for your particular specialty and department with input from all staff members. At the same time, it is helpful to hear from Primary Nurses in different organizations and to learn what is working for them. We will share what has worked well for many of them in accomplishing the following:

- Effective assignment of patients.

- Introducing oneself and explaining the Primary Nursing role to patients and families.

- Effective ways of integrating associate nurses into the Primary Nursing care delivery system.

- Optimizing the electronic medical record (EMR) to support Primary Nursing.

- Facilitating communication with people in other disciplines.

- Heading off the emotional toll of working with high-acuity patients.

- Continually adapting systems and processes that support Primary Nursing.

- Getting the initial buy-in of the team.

Individual interviews were conducted with seasoned Primary Nurses from inpatient, perioperative, and ambulatory settings. They are passionate about the positive impact this care delivery system has had on their patients and on their sense of personal fulfillment as professional nurses.

We were not surprised to find that when these Primary Nurses worked to design and refine the changes that would be necessary in their work processes and systems, they did so with patients and families in mind. We were struck, however, by the specificity of this commitment. The systems and processes these nurses and their interdisciplinary colleagues designed and refined in order to make Primary Nursing a way of thinking, being, and doing in their departments were designed around the specifics of their patient populations. In at least one case, those designing the system of Primary Nursing surveyed their patients to find out what they valued most about their current care, so they could tailor their systems and processes to remove all barriers to the nurses doing more of those things, and they looked at what their patients told them was not working as well, so they could refine their infrastructure and practices to address the gaps they discovered.

For the convenience of the reader, the voices of each of the nurses interviewed were organized into topic areas, and some have been edited for clarity. A list of these exemplary individuals and their organizations can be found in the Acknowledgments on page xi. We are extraordinarily grateful for the wisdom, insight, and passion they've offered in service to the readers of this book and, by extension, to all of the patients and families our readers will touch.

Systems of Assignment That Promote Nurse–Patient Continuity

A variety of methods of assignments were effective for the nurses we interviewed. In every case, however, the method of assignment evolved over time as part of the continuous improvement of the systems they built. It was clear that systems that best served patients and families on some units were ultimately not in the best interest of patients and families on others.

EXAMPLE 1

We divided our 50+ nurses into four color teams—red, blue, green, and yellow—on our 34-bed hematology/oncology unit. We divided the teams as evenly as we could based on seniority, preceptors, charge capability, and a balance of day and night nurses. Each color team included a member of our Relationship-Based Care council to help with communication. When a patient is admitted, the admitting nurse is the Primary Nurse; that nurse notifies the charge nurse and puts his or her name in the EMR. The charge nurse is not only doing assignments to ensure continuity but also following up on admissions to make sure that the admitting nurse is assigned as a Primary Nurse. The most pivotal person in making this system of assignment successful is the charge nurse. From the beginning we created an algorithm for assignments, and this really helped make sure every patient has a Primary Nurse and that associate nurses are from the same color team. The way our charge nurses make the assignments is to first see if there's anyone coming in who has a primary patient. If not, they look for members on the same color team that they can assign to this patient. We do make allowances for acuity. We wouldn't give someone four heavy-acuity patients just because they're red; we make sure it makes sense. After that, we look at who can care for the patient the next day.

EXAMPLE 2

We've been doing Primary Nursing since 1997 on our pediatric unit. Initially there were a lot of guidelines and we had color groups. There was always a Primary Nurse, whether it was the first nurse who admitted the patient or another nurse who connected with them. The patient became part of that color group. Later as the EMR was implemented, colors sort of faded away. We had the opportunity to sign up as the Primary Nurse or associate nurse. All patients receive a Primary Nurse within the first 24 or 36 hours. It's all based on the charge nurse assigning the patient, and they have the criteria. We aren't holding to it having to be the admitting nurse, but rather the first person who has a chance to build a rapport with them. With the computer system, we were able to save the names and stay consistent for future admissions.

EXAMPLE 3

In perioperative services, once the patient arrives in pre-op, we assign the Primary Nurse there. The pre-op nurse remains the Primary Nurse throughout the perioperative experience. That nurse spends maybe an hour with the patient and can establish the relationship. We tried other ways, but patients couldn't remember the OR nurse or recovery nurse because of the anesthesia, so this works best.

EXAMPLE 4

Our ambulatory clinic is multifunctional, with things like exam clinic, infusions, nurse practitioner clinic, labs, education, and so forth. We identified one overall Primary Nurse rather than one for each function. Each Primary Nurse is linked with a primary doctor and that doctor's roster of patients. There is a team that consists of the primary physician, nurse practitioner, Primary Nurse, and associate nurse. It works really wonderfully in our clinic.

EXAMPLE 5

Our floor has 12-hour shifts. Once a nurse has been here 6 months he or she can be a Primary Nurse. We match the Primary Nurse with an associate nurse. You can sign up to be an associate after meeting the patient, often when the Primary Nurse is off. That way when the Primary Nurse is not working, the associate nurse has a high chance of having the patient. When we do assignments, the first priority is to give everyone their Primary Nurse, then who was here yesterday, then give everyone their associates. We do all of our assignments based on Primary Nursing, and the charge nurse for the prior shift will print out a list; it's easy to do. After many years we gave up the color system. It wasn't a bad system; we probably used color groups for 10 years, but after going to the EMR we realized it took work to maintain colors without much benefit. We had to deal with "crossover" patients, assigned to another color team on another admission. Even though we tried to visit them, really the families drove the change since they wanted the same Primary Nurse.

Example 6

We realized that it took work to maintain the color system with very little benefit. We're nurses, so we like our boxes, colors, teams, etc., which give the illusion of order. In small ways it hurt rather than helped our overall goal, which was, "What does this patient and family think is best, and what does the Primary Nurse think is best for this family?"

> *We're nurses, so we like our boxes, colors, teams, etc., which give the illusion of order.*

Example 7

When we started, because we didn't fully know what we were doing, we didn't assign new grads for the first year out of orientation, so for the first year of their nursing they had no primary patients. Now that so many of us are entrenched in it, we assign them primary patients. They might not yet know what early signs of sepsis look like, but since they know their patients, they are able to identify that something is wrong more quickly. They say they're getting the bigger picture faster.

Introduction and Explanation of the Primary Nursing Role to the Patient and Family

Experience has shown that the introduction by a Primary Nurse to the patient is very important in establishing the relationship. The language used is important in conveying the commitment inherent in Primary Nursing. Best practice is that somewhere in that introduction, the Primary Nurse should say the words, "I am your Primary Nurse." These words convey to both the nurse and to the patient that he or she has accepted the responsibility for serving in this role.

Many organizations have established letters or cards that can be given to supplement (but not replace) the verbal introduction. These cards or letters reinforce both the name of the Primary Nurse and the fact that the Primary Nurse has taken responsibility for being the patient's and family's go-to source of information, comfort, and advocacy. Here are samples of verbal introductions from experienced Primary Nurses.

EXAMPLE 1

We say something like, "I'm your Primary Nurse, and what that means is that ideally every time you're here, I'm here helping take care of you. I'll advocate for you, I'll be your point of communication, I'll be support for you and your family, and I'll answer any questions you have. In case I'm not here, someone in our color group will take care of you." There is no set script; we all personalize it.

EXAMPLE 2

Initially the biggest challenge was to get people to say, "I am your Primary Nurse"—just to get the verbiage out. I don't understand why that was difficult for nurses to do in the beginning, but now it's easy. Some of our patients have memory issues. When I'm their Primary Nurse, I continue to tell them and tell them until they can ask for me by name or say "hi" to me by name. They don't always realize how important it is for them to be able to ask for me by name, but I do. I know that if they get disoriented or worried about something, they're going to be glad they know the name of the person who knows them and their condition best.

> *I know that if they get disoriented or worried about something, they're going to be glad they know the name of the person who knows them and their condition best.*

EXAMPLE 3

Once I sign up as a Primary Nurse, and once everyone is settled in (not during the welcome to the hospital speech), I explain Primary Nursing. If I'm not quite sure we've made a connection I might explain that they have the option of having me as their Primary Nurse. I explain the role, adding that as long as you're here and I'm here, I will be caring for you. I tell them that I'll also work with their other nurses when I'm not here, communicating what your preferences are, what your needs are, in the hope that it will give you more consistent care no matter how long you're here. Across the board, that just always gets a collective exhale from the families no matter why they're here.

Actions That Reinforce the Primary Nurse Role for Patients and Families

While the verbal introduction to Primary Nursing is absolutely vital, many additional actions can reinforce how much of a lifeline the Primary Nurse can be to patients and families. It's important to remember also that Primary Nursing will be completely new to most patients and families, so it is helpful to orient them over and over to the practice and what it can mean to them.

ACTION 1

If I'm here and I find out that any of my primary patients are in today, I'll make it a point to go talk to them to really reinforce the primary relationship. I just want to make them feel more comfortable, make sure I'm giving them holistic care—not just worrying about their physical health, but addressing their mental and emotional health. We find out through our audits that patients realize we care; we communicate, we take the time to listen and explain things.

ACTION 2

We have it set up so that we can go and see our patients on their units after surgery. It gives the OR nurse a connection because we get a chance to say, "I took care of you for ten hours … but you didn't really know it." So again that's building the relationship.

ACTION 3

We redesigned the whiteboards in our patient rooms to have a specific place for the Primary Nurse as well as the nurse of the day. We also tend to say the name of the Primary Nurse during bedside shift report to reinforce who that is and that we are communicating. We also added spaces for Primary Therapists and so forth.

ACTION 4

During surgery, patients move through lots of different areas, so we created a Primary Nurse passport, a small tent card made of cardboard. It has the name of the Primary Nurse and all the other caregivers listed. This passport goes with them through all phases of care, like OR and recovery room. It contains personal information, such as answers to questions like, "What questions or priorities do you have?" This allows everyone to learn some important things about the patient. It fulfills part of the role of the Primary Nurse to learn about the patient as a person and what is important to them.

Role and Importance of Associate Nurses

As in most of the design of Primary Nursing, the ways in which associate nurses are integrated will be customized based on what best supports the continuity of patient–caregiver assignments. There is flexibility in how best to use associate nurses to maintain a consistent relationship and clinical care when the Primary Nurse is not present. This can range from designating an associate nurse to work opposite shifts from the Primary Nurse and having another one on the same shift to cover the Primary Nurse's days off, as well as many other combinations. Your council should decide what works best for your department, with the caveat that your system for assignment of associates must result in patients experiencing the fewest possible different caregivers.

EXAMPLE 1

Associate nurses are very helpful, especially between shifts. Some staff members felt that very complex patients shouldn't have a Primary Nurse who works nights. My manager decided not to get in the middle of that decision—not to say who could or couldn't be a Primary Nurse. If the night nurse is the Primary Nurse, there is an unofficial agreement with the day shift nurse about picking up the communication slack, being a strong associate on days to support the night Primary Nurse. Some people said there should just be two primaries, but my manager has drawn a hard line in saying that having two Primaries would completely defeat the purpose of Primary Nursing. Instead, we get a really strong associate.

Example 2

With our color groups, having just a few associate nurses wasn't really feasible. Any member of the same color group can function as an associate, and camaraderie is strong within the groups. We have high continuity of assignments when the Primary Nurse is not there.

Use of the Electronic Medical Record to Support Primary Nursing

Use of the EMR strongly facilitates smooth handoffs and seamless care, and it enables the Primary Nurse to efficiently convey personal information, preferences, and the plan of care to everyone who cares for that patient.

Example 1

When we first got the EMR, we were taught that if something had been on a paper Kardex, it would now be on the "sticky note" part of the EMR. It would not stay, and did not have to be perfectly written, since it was not a permanent record. It's a place to record something that's pertinent right now. Doctors, nurses, physical therapists, anybody ... when they open the patient's chart, it's the front screen that you see, so people from other services have the opportunity to set themselves up for success if they read the Primary Nurse communications. When I'm training residents, I let them know that if they ever find out more information about the patient, just press this button and add the information to the sticky note and set me up for success as well. Otherwise, the patient can say, "Gosh, I've said that 500 times; why does nobody know that I don't like apple juice?"

Example 2

When we become the Primary Nurse, we establish the relationship with the patient and then in the EMR we'll put in what they call a snapshot in communication. This is where we can see all the Primary Nurses throughout the hospital for this patient from when they were cared for in other departments or clinics.

Example 3

In our EMR, every patient has a treatment team—their attending physician, usually their admitting physician, and then what you can do is add yourself as the Primary Nurse or associate nurse. That information follows them through every admission so that when they are readmitted, as long as they're in our system, anyone can click in and see who serves in each role. They will have a Primary Nurse in ICU, a Primary Nurse on the floor, and even a Primary in the infusion room.

Example 4

For our clinic, when a patient is discharged from the hospital, the inpatient department will route us a message through the EMR to let us know that the patient has been discharged. Then we can do the post-discharge follow-up call and appointment. If our clinic patient needs to be admitted, the charge nurse may call to the unit that will likely get the patient so they can prepare to assign the Primary Nurse. We are doing more and more with that communication loop between the hospital and clinic. If we have put our name in the EMR as part of the care team, when that referring physician puts a note in, we automatically get a message about what happened at that visit.

Interdisciplinary and Handover Communication

Primary Nursing elevates the professional status of nurses as equal members of the professional care team. This goes far beyond a "nurse of the day" standing in for patient rounds or an interdisciplinary conference. The Primary Nurse is able to more knowledgeably and confidently advocate for the patient, communicate his or her progress and preferences, and offer recommendations to the physician for needed orders.

Example 1

In our charting we have a Primary Nurse communication section. We have found that it's keeping track of the small, patient-based things that really helps. A parent may say, "Wow, you already know that my daughter likes chocolate syrup with her medicines."

EXAMPLE 2

I think the biggest thing we can do as the Primary Nurse is to help with the verbal communication, because otherwise so much is lost. We can help empower families to communicate and to know what questions to ask and help everybody know what the plan is. If families have a Primary Nurse or a group of interdisciplinary people as their primary team who are willing to advocate for them, families will feel that, and we definitely see it show up on patient satisfaction surveys.

EXAMPLE 3

In perioperative services, based on our CREW and Relationship-Based Care initiatives, we created a pre-op-to-OR handoff communication tool. The pre-op nurse and the OR nurse go through the communication handoff tool in front of the patient. What we tell the patient is, "We're going to go over your plan of care in front of you. Please let us know if there's anything additional, if there's anything that we left out, or if you have any concerns." And that really helps with our patient satisfaction because we really get to know the patient, and their family is better informed and can be partners. After surgery we have a sign-out debriefing in the OR. Each person is asked what went well, and what are some red flags we need to tell PACU? Is there anything that didn't go well? Sometimes concerns are equipment related, but it's all about the patient—what went well, what we could have done better. We developed this as a tool with CREW resource management, and were lucky that we got it before Primary Nursing kicked off. After we do our debrief and sign out and wake the patient up, we call in a report on the phone; then we bring the patient to PACU and do a handoff report in person.

EXAMPLE 4

We're unique in how many services come through our unit, so often the role of the Primary Nurse is to serve as a kind of communications wrangler to get everybody on the same page, to encourage the setting up of family meetings, and to do something we jokingly call "nag-vocating." We Primary Nurses end up nag-vocating for our patients all the time. We have to respect the learning environment as a teaching hospital and still keep a safe and open place for families, helping explain and translate what is going on.

Example 5

In our clinic we do have a triage role, and we integrated it into Primary Nursing. If one of my colleagues takes a call from one of my primary patients who is having issues, the constant communication is important. So, the triage nurse works to coordinate care at that time of need, but then opens up a telephone encounter to document the issues. We can route the messages to the Primary Nurse and team. This addition has helped keep the Primary Nurse in the loop. If you as Primary Nurse return the next day you can follow up and see what was effective.

At times, the value of the Primary Nurse as a collector, holder, and transmitter of important information about the patient is incalculable, as in the following example.

Example 6

Primary Nursing really gives a voice to a lot of patients who wouldn't be able to speak up for themselves. We have a lot of kids with cerebral palsy who are in protective custody or foster care because of abuse, and their Primary Nurse is able to make sure that the docs are in the know. Maybe the social worker is coming off of vacation—the Primary Nurse makes sure that everybody knows what this kid needs, what their baselines look like, and what the possible traps and vulnerabilities are for kids with no parents.

When Patient Care Takes an Emotional Toll

The care of some patients and families can be challenging for reasons ranging from acuity of the patient's condition to abusiveness of the patient and/or family or even to the personal circumstances of the nurses themselves. The improved collegial relationships on units in which Primary Nursing is practiced can be a huge benefit when care gets heavy.

EXAMPLE 1

The role of associate nurses is even more important when patients or families are challenging in some way. If the Primary Nurse needs a night off from that assignment, give it to them. With certain families we learned early on that we needed to watch the Primary Nurse for signs of burnout. If that happens, assign them to other patients. Make sure you "spread the wealth." It's easy to say, "Give the tough situations to those four nurses who can handle it," but we are really moving away from that mentality. Peer support has been important for these situations. And empowering our new grads—telling them that these aren't people to shy away from—is something we're starting to do more consistently. Committing to these families as Primary Nurses is a step toward figuring out how to give these families the same quality of care we give to everyone else.

EXAMPLE 2

Several years ago, two friends and my grandparents all died within several months of each other, and I had nine patients, who were very close to me who I'd taken care of for a very long time, all pass within that same 6 or 8 month period. The bounce-back from that came very slowly before I could comfortably be a Primary Nurse for a complex patient. And without my even being aware of it, my manager, assistant manager, and the relief charge nurses, knowing that all of these losses had been going on for me, only gave me kids with broken bones, kids with diabetes, kids with tonsillitis, kids with appendicitis, and the occasional more complex patient. I didn't even realize they'd been deliberately giving me the less complex patients until a year had passed; then I realized that I wasn't as terrified of going in to work as I had been. It's difficult to quantify because it's very intuitive on my floor, how it's done, the care of each nurse.

EXAMPLE 3

We have a lot of challenging socioeconomic situations, and sometimes it would be easier not to care for a patient because they're hard. But they're probably the ones who need Primary Nursing more than the easy ones, because they need consistency, and they need guidance. They really need to be heard and understood.

Be Ready to Adapt Continually

On units doing Primary Nursing, it's important to keep measuring impact, to keep an eye on outcomes, and to always feel free to make changes after a reasonable trial. The electronic medical record (EMR) is a classic example of a catalyst for sitting down to consider adaptations to the way Primary Nursing works on your unit. As a new initiative, it will create new challenges and opportunities. It can be exceptionally gratifying to figure out how to meet challenges and maximize opportunities in order to provide the best possible care. However, even without a catalyst, there is great benefit to periodically assessing and adapting the way Primary Nursing works on your unit. No matter what decision or change you make, just make sure everyone does it the same way so that you can really tell whether the system is not working or people are just not working within the system.

EXAMPLE 1

I think the most important thing to keep in mind is to be adaptable. If you see obstacles or opportunities, bring them up to your manager. Be sure to speak up, even if things are running smoothly; it's easy to dismiss good ideas because you think they're not possible.

EXAMPLE 2

If something's not working, we make a change, and we use our audit results to decide what to work on. I'll admit that in the last few months, we've gotten a little stagnant, because we thought, "This is working; this is good," but we see also that we have to constantly work on it because it's a living, breathing thing. Getting stuck in the idea that whatever you created is "it" is going to get you stuck because you really do have to adapt and change.

Getting Buy-in from the Team

Resistance to Primary Nursing is often due to the way it is presented to the group. This is a time for thoughtfulness and subtlety. The following examples demonstrate the best of both.

Example 1

There were two really key moments in the development of how Primary Nursing was going to look on our unit, and the first one was when we sat down and looked at everything that *wasn't* going to work— all of the current barriers—and we really focused on that. We were looking at all of our current initiatives and worrying about things like, "How are people going to accept this on top of everything else?" and "Look at all of these obstacles: such a large unit, staffing that didn't seem ideal for it ..." We decided to be "realistic."

And then one day we decided instead to sit down and figure out, in an ideal world, what would Primary Nursing look like for us? We also decided that we didn't need to reinvent the wheel. We decided to look at what we have and look at what it *could* be, and then just map it out. We decided to forget all of our obstacles and just see what we *can* do. From that point on the whole dynamic of the group changed, and we got so many more ideas. It's so easy to get focused on the obstacles and what may not work, and once you remove those mental barriers, it was exciting and we could see the vision. Before that, it was right in front of us, but we couldn't see it because we were focused on the barriers. That was really a turning point for us.

> *Focus your energy on the people who will get excited, because positivity breeds positivity.*

The second piece to that was, I think people are just drawn to focusing on the negative aspects. Again we were wondering, "How are we going to sell this to our staff?" We started thinking about the five or six people who we knew would be a really hard sell—that's who we were focusing on when we were trying to come up with our staff presentation. All of a sudden, Jennifer gave us this idea: She challenged us to think instead of the people who are sure to get excited about this. Focus your energy on the people who will get excited, because positivity breeds positivity. And we changed our whole focus again. When we did our presentation to the staff we really focused on those who were excited. We still had issues, there were questions and concerns to address and follow up on, and there were still naysayers, but now, even those who were a hard sell in the beginning have come to really be part of it in their own way.

Example 2

One of our nurses shared her stories about what it meant to her to be a Primary Nurse. We're all so compassionate here that no one could hear these stories and say, "No, I don't want to do Primary Nursing." We talked about the bond with patients and how important we are in their entire care plan. I don't know anyone who sat there and said, "No I don't want to do that." Maybe some thought they didn't want to do it quite the way it was presented, but everyone thought, "That's cool; I'd like to have that." Actually hearing what it meant to other people—how I can benefit—that's the biggest thing.

Example 3

I think the key factor in getting buy-in is to make sure everyone is involved. With any kind of change there will be resistance, so it's important to involve your patients. We also involved our schedulers, and we involved our PCAs/nursing assistants. That way everybody feels like a team; everybody on the unit feels involved. It's definitely true that when we were rolling this out, some other changes were also going on, which brings even more resistance to change, so getting everybody involved, getting everybody's input and making sure that you're visibly incorporating it, really helped.

Example 4

When something is being done for patient safety, it's a "have to"—period. So once we implemented Primary Nursing we gave lots of reasons. We really told them why. We gave the data and patient comments. Sharing evidence that it's working is a really a good way to get staff to buy in.

Example 5

Early on I think Primary Nursing was looked at as another thing we had to do, but once we found out that we got to own it, people take a lot more pride and responsibility for something they get to own and create versus something they have pushed upon them. Then, being an outpatient unit, with no real evidence available for how it could work—even that it could be done on outpatient—maybe it made us work even harder at it. You're going to be the first: lead the way.

Questions for Reflection

- In your department or a department you know well, what sort of patient assignment system might work best? If you've seen a system of assignment work well within a department that practices Primary Nursing, reflect on and share what you know about that system.

- Why is it important to make sure the patient and family know the name of their Primary Nurse?

- How important is handoff communication in health care in general? What are some of the most patient-centric ways you've experienced or heard about to handle handoffs?

- Share some examples of highly effective interdisciplinary collaboration you have experienced. What made them effective, particularly in terms of the role of the nurse?

Primary Nursing provides the framework for building a trusting relationship for both the nurse and the patient, thus supporting optimal healing and health.

Judy Blauwet, RN, BSN, MPH, FACHE, NE-BC
Sr. VP of Hospital Operations/CNO, Avera McKennan Hospital
Avera McKennan Nursing received its fourth consecutive
Magnet designation in 2015

Chapter 9

Care Team Partners in Primary Nursing

One of the hallmarks of the Primary Nursing role is the clarity with which RNs accept responsibility for decision making regarding the care of the patient. It is the unique role and responsibility of registered nurses that they are licensed to determine the kind and amount of nursing care the patient needs and how much of that care can be delegated to other caregivers (Koloroutis, 2004).

The Primary Nurse determines and prioritizes the needs of the patient and family in order to establish an individualized plan of care. Some of that care may be delegated to associate nurses, LPNs, nursing assistants, nursing technicians, and other caregivers. There is a need to clearly differentiate the practice of RNs and LPNs and to be consistent with state Nurse Practice Acts. Primary Nursing provides clarity of roles and important gains related to consistent relationships.

Providing the structure for how caregivers relate to each other is a critical and complex responsibility of leadership. RNs are often working in isolation, not getting or giving assistance. The need for paired or partnered relationships that Marie Manthey first identified in the 1980s (Manthey, 1989) continues to be a strategy that brings caregivers into collaborative practice and that supports role clarity and appropriate delegation (Forstrom & Weydt, 2008).

Advantages of Assignments Using Pairs or Partners

Direct caregivers who work together consistently, experience the following gains in the work setting:

- Increased efficiency in getting the work done through natural synergy (staff members report a 25% reduction in workload and stress).

- More knowledge about each other's competence, a foundation for delegation.

- Opportunities for continued learning and advancement of partner skills.

- Better communication within the team and among other shifts and departments (more than 50% of sentinel events are related to communication errors).

- Increased commitment to each other and the ability to deal with more complex situations (vital behaviors for effective work teams in high-acuity care settings).

To demonstrate these advantages, we can consider three methods of making assignments when using assistive personnel in the clinical setting. There are advantages and disadvantages to each.

- **Unit-based assignments** occur when assistants serve most or all RNs on the unit rather than getting directions from one or two individuals. Usually the assistants carry out the same work activities each day, as if they own the work rather than the RN having overall responsibility for it. An example is measuring and recording the vital signs for all patients on the floor, a task-based rather than a patient-centered activity. In this scenario, RNs may not be thinking critically about whether they should take vital signs on some patients.

- **Pairing** is defined as one RN working with a nursing assistant, LPN, technician, or other care assistant. This pair works with each other for this shift but not necessarily for future shifts.

- **Partnering** is defined as one RN consistently working with another specific caregiver. The two work together by choice, coordinating their schedules when possible. They make a commitment to maintain a healthy interpersonal relationship, recognizing that the RN has the authority to make the delegation decisions. They commit to advancing each other's knowledge.

In both paired and partnered assignments, team members see the patients as their joint responsibility and make the most of one another's contributions in the interest of patient care. For example, if there is a bath to do, there is no mandate on a care team that either team member always does baths if both team members possess the knowledge, skill, and licensure to do the work. The decision is based on the best way to meet patient needs in a timely manner. In pairing and partnering, the team members care for "our" patients rather than "yours" and "mine"—a major shift in thinking and in how assignments and care decisions are made.

The care team partnership arrangement is the more intentional, consistent relationship and offers the best solution to the highly variable and inconsistent patient–nurse relationships so common in today's acute care environments. There can be times when care team partners are not working together, but that is the exception, not the rule. Vacations, floating, illnesses, and other situations may interrupt the partnership, but the partnership is stable enough that the partners learn each other's special talents and work preferences, communicate more effectively, and provide for each other's growth. In this way, teamwork and trust are enhanced. This intentional team is positioned to provide patients and families with care that is more compassionate, competent, and clinically and emotionally safe. As Marie wrote more than a decade ago:

> The utilization of auxiliary personnel needs to be done in a partnership or a paired system. Then we don't have people running around doing a lot of tasks, but rather we incorporate them into a holistic perspective of care for a group of patients under the direction of a knowledgeable RN. (Manthey, 2002)

Delegation Principles

Historically, the confusion about roles and responsibilities, particularly those of RNs and LPNs, has contributed to LPNs being assigned beyond the scope of their licensure as well as delegation decisions that are task-based rather than knowledge-based.

It is helpful to remember that although RNs are responsible for their decisions about what to delegate, they are not responsible for the faultless performance of the delegee. Delegees are responsible for their own actions.

RNs are responsible for using good judgment when delegating and for increasing the effectiveness of delegation by:

- Understanding the scope of practice of RNs, LPNs, and other assistants.

- Matching the work to the knowledge and skills of the delegee. The person delegating should have no reason to believe that the delegee cannot carry out the work safely and effectively.

- Providing timely data and instruction to the delegee (giving appropriate information about the patient, the priority, expected timelines, how the work needs to be done, and situations in which the delegee should immediately report information to the RN).

- Being available to answer questions from the delegee.

- Ensuring that the work has been completed in a timely and effective manner through appropriate follow-up. (Forstrom & Weydt, 2008)

Trust and mutual respect can develop when care partners are valued as team members, when their observations and input are solicited, and when their feelings about the work environment are sought and appreciated.

Remembering the five rights of delegation can serve as a helpful tool when making delegation decisions.

Five Rights of Delegation

1. Right Task

2. Right Circumstances

3. Right Person

4. Right Direction/Communication

5. Right Supervision/Evaluation (National Council of State Boards of Nursing, 2005)

It is our opinion—one that is supported by evidence-based practice—that the plan for implementation of Primary Nursing should include a system for assigning staff members in partnerships whenever possible. The advantages will be felt by both patients and team members (Wessel, Felgen, Person, & Kinnaird, 2008).

Summary of Key Points

- Primary Nursing provides clarity of roles and important gains related to consistent relationships.

- Direct caregivers who work together consistently, experience increased efficiency, more opportunities for continued learning and advancement of partner skills, and better communication within the team and among other shifts and departments. They are also better able to handle complex situations as a team and have more knowledge about one another's competence.

- In both paired and partnered assignments, team members see the patients as their joint responsibility and make the most of one another's contributions in the interest of patient care.

- When working in paired or partnered assignments, although RNs are responsible for their decisions about what to delegate, they are not responsible for the faultless performance of the delegee. Delegees are responsible for their own actions.

Questions for Reflection

- Think about or discuss the benefits of maintaining consistent teams of caregivers.

- Compare and contrast paired assignments and partnered assignments until you can articulate the difference.

I remember when we started this journey, I had only done team nursing, and the Primary Nurses who had done it before would tear up when they would talk about it. I love my primary patients. When there are admitted on other floors, I go see them; I see them in the ICU. We really care about our primary patients because we form such a close bond with them.

KIRSTEN ROBLEE, BSN, RN, OCN
PRIMARY NURSE AT OSUCCC—JAMES

Chapter 10

Best Practices in Sustaining and Deepening Primary Nursing

Best Practices for Keeping Primary Nursing Strong

When Primary Nursing is supported and consciously reinforced, it can be a powerful way to develop professional practice in newer nurses and to strengthen it in experienced nurses. This is best accomplished with reflection and sharing. When nurses are asked regularly to identify the most important nursing problems and interventions they used with patients, they become more conscious about the important critical thinking and decisions they are making as part of the nursing process. Certainly the regular use of case conferences is a fundamental way to keep Primary Nursing alive, and there are less formal daily practices that help as well.

As managers, educators, or preceptors make informal rounds with staff, the use of reflective questions to stimulate a nurse's thought process can be very effective. Here are a few examples of questions that reinforce the independent role of professional nurses (choose one or two rather than several; your aim is to inspire, not to interrogate):

- For which patients are you Primary Nurse right now? Tell me about one of them.

- What are the most important nursing problems (or nursing diagnoses) you have identified?

- Share the most important nursing interventions you're providing this patient and how the patient is responding.

- What side effects or complications are you keeping an eye out for?

- What have you learned about your primary patient and family that has allowed you to personalize their care?

- What suggestions, if any, are you planning to make to the physician?

- What other disciplines or services have you involved to help with the care of this patient?

- What are you proud of regarding the care you have provided as the Primary Nurse for this patient?

In addition to reflection, nurses should be encouraged to use every opportunity to remind the patient of the name of the Primary Nurse and to reinforce the Primary Nurse's role. Examples may include:

- Recording the name of the Primary Nurse (and primary caregivers from other disciplines) on a whiteboard. (See Appendix D for an example.)

- Conducting a brief survey as the patient is leaving to determine whether the patient knows the name of his or her Primary Nurse; this is an important component in assessing the effectiveness of the relationship. (See Appendix H for an example.)

- Using shift report or interdisciplinary rounds as an opportunity to reinforce the role and significance of the Primary Nurse and the patient–nurse relationship.

- Offering the patient and/or family a letter or business card upon arrival which includes the name of the Primary Nurse and a description of the role.

- When follow-up phone calls are made, have them made by the Primary Nurse whenever possible.

When nursing care for a complex patient is particularly effective, consider having the Primary Nurse share a brief case presentation following discharge or transfer (see p. 85). This encourages learning and the sharing of best practices among practitioners, which is especially helpful for newer nurses.

Best Manager Strategies for Sustaining and Reinforcing Primary Nursing

- Continue to ensure regular meetings of your UPC (at least monthly), arranging coverage as possible. The council may take on a broader function, but part of their role should remain the continuous improvement of Primary Nursing.

- Attend a portion of each UPC meeting. Often staff members will state a preferred time and length for your participation. When you are unable to attend, meet with the chair within a week after the meeting for an update and to ask what they need from you.

- Use staff meetings to state explicitly that you support and appreciate the plan for Primary Nursing developed by council members. Convey your expectation that everyone in the unit or department follow the plan and let you know anything they might need to succeed. In particular, state that you believe that Primary Nursing will take the quality of care to a higher level and help staff feel even more satisfied in their work.

- Make the UPC report a standing item on the agenda for staff meetings to share the newest outcome measures and any reminders that will help fully implement the plan.

- During performance appraisal meetings, ask staff members, "Tell me about a patient for whom you were a Primary Nurse and how you made a positive difference through your relationship." Or ask, "Share an example of a patient for whom your decisions about their care really made a positive difference." Or, "In what ways has Primary Nursing enhanced interdisciplinary collaboration?"

- Begin staff meetings with a Primary Nursing story, rotating the specifics:

  » Read a patient letter that includes a moving description of meaningful care.

  » Share a comment related to their Primary Nurse made by a patient/family member when you made rounds.

  » Share a comment made by a patient when you made rounds complimenting the care provided by a tech or nursing assistant.

  » Ask someone to share a success story in caring for a primary patient with special or complex response/needs (anger, anxiety, confusion, being withdrawn, etc.).

  » Ask someone to share a success story in collaborating with a physician that really benefited a patient.

- When making patient rounds, after you introduce yourself, ask questions such as, "What has your care been like for you?" Then explore their answer in more depth. "Who is your Primary Nurse?" "Has your Primary Nurse helped you through a difficult situation? Tell me about that." "What could we do to improve your care?" "Is there someone you'd like me to recognize who has helped you?"

- Ask physicians for an example of a Primary Nurse who made a positive difference for one of their patients. Ask how the staff could be even more helpful in supporting clinicians providing medical care. Ask how collaboration and/or collegiality have strengthened since the implementation of Primary Nursing.

- Attend the Steering Council or other management meetings with your UPC chair and help him or her prepare for sharing your unit's most current outcome measures.

We have seen, time and again, that the manager's commitment to Primary Nursing makes all the difference in whether it is sustained and flourishes or fades. A commitment to Primary Nursing must begin with a strong vision and ongoing recognition, encouragement, and reinforcement by the chief nurse executive.

We began to understand that the underlying principles of Primary Nursing were more than the design of a nursing assignment or delivery system. They represented the conceptual framework for professional nursing practice.

JOYCE C. CLIFFORD, RN, PHD, FAAN
PRIMARY NURSING PIONEER

Epilogue:

The Message Behind the Words, "I Am Your Primary Nurse"

A patient in an outpatient surgery center shared an experience that reinforced the importance of having a Primary Nurse, the one nurse who says, "I am here, and I will take care of you."

Marietta described her nurse, Theresa, as "friendly and somewhat reassuring," yet something was missing. "She either didn't pick up on my nervousness, or she didn't want to take the time to find out what was going on with me." After asking Marietta a few questions related to her condition, Theresa said, "You work at the hospital don't you? You look familiar." Marietta told her that she did work at the hospital. It seemed for a moment that Theresa was making an attempt to get to know Marietta, but she dropped the topic as quickly as it arose; it was nothing more than idle chitchat. For Theresa, everything was routine, just another day; she had no connection to Marietta's fear and need for reassurance. In recapping the subtle uneasiness she'd felt with Theresa, Marietta said, "No one asked me why I didn't want sedation. They just moved forward without really partnering with me, saying, 'Dr. Right is a calming presence; reassuring. No sedation is a good choice; you'll be able to go about your day.' I got exactly what I asked for, so I'm not sure why I'm complaining. ... I guess it just felt like I was in it alone."

Marietta went on to say that everything was explained to her, and she didn't feel rushed, but she described the interactions with her health care providers as not feeling seen, as though she didn't really matter. After interacting with four people (the registration clerk, two nurses, and a nursing assistant), Marietta noticed, "No one asked, 'How are you?'—at least not in a way that felt like they actually wanted to know." There was no inquiry about whether anything was concerning her or any interaction that made her feel as though she was a unique human being. Rather, she described feeling that she was receiving the exact same care anyone would receive; there was no individualization to meet her unique needs.

Finally, Marietta met Sara, who said, "I'll be your Primary Nurse during your procedure. I'll be with you the entire time, and I will make sure you're safe and that all of your questions get answered." Imagine an exhale so full and deep that it makes you suddenly aware of the extent to which you've been holding your breath. Marietta experienced a change from feeling as though she was part of somebody's workload to feeling seen as a human being. Sara took responsibility and let Marietta know it, and with that act—a simple act of "holding"—everything changed for Marietta.

Many of the nurses we work with are reticent at first to say, "I am responsible." "I will take care of you." "I am your Primary Nurse." There is something daunting about singling yourself out and stepping up as the one who commits to making a difference. And yet there really is no substitute. When you put yourself in the patient's shoes, it becomes clear that "I will take care of you" means everything, and *"we* will take care of you" is a nice neutral phrase indicating that nobody whose name you know or whose number you have has made a commitment to really watching out for you.

In a 2009 address to the International Forum on Quality and Safety in Health Care, former Administrator of the Centers for Medicare and Medicaid Services Don Berwick spoke to this reality quite clearly:

> What chills my bones [about the thought of being a patient] is indignity. It is the loss of influence on what happens to me. It is the image of myself in a hospital gown, homogenized, anonymous, powerless, no longer myself. It is the sound of a young nurse calling me "Donald" which is a name I never use—It's Don. It is the voice of the doctor saying "We think," instead of "I think," and thereby placing that small verbal wedge, the pronoun "we," between himself as a person and myself as a person. (Berwick, 2009)

In health care, the word "we" provides little comfort for patients and families. "We will take care of you" means that a large, nameless, faceless collection of people (or an institution) accepts some degree of responsibility for your wellbeing. If you are a patient or a concerned family member, you are probably aware that if "they" are largely anonymous to you, you are almost certainly anonymous to them. You want someone to step up and say, "I will be responsible for partnering with you, to learn what is important to you. I will make sure you understand the plan for you, and I will communicate what you and I agree on to others caring for you so your care will be consistent. Because I'm your Primary Nurse, everyone who cares for you will know what's important to you."

Stepping into the formidable role of "I" can be a significant barrier to nurses who are new to Primary Nursing. There is often an initial reluctance to claim that level of responsibility. But that reluctance goes away over time and is replaced by a real appreciation for the autonomy it brings. Heidi Nolen, Primary Nurse at UC Davis, sees it this way:

> I think that until they've had the experience of being a Primary Nurse, they worry about it—just the fear of the unknown. But as soon as they have the experience, they see how it benefits the patient and family and themselves as nurses. It's just really special, and they might not really get it until they have that aha experience, when they realize, "Oh, now I know what you were saying! I really fell in love with that family, or I really felt great about myself that I was able to get that kid what he needed to get out of the hospital." Or fighting a battle for them that only you could fight because you really know them. There are so many ways you can have that aha moment, but until you do, it's a little scary.

Surely, the notion of responsibility can be daunting. And yet, while it is very common in departments new to Primary Nursing for nurses to resist accepting responsibility at first, it is equally common, once Primary Nursing is fully implemented in the department, for Primary Nurses to become staunch defenders of this care delivery system. If you give people a taste of high-quality Primary Nursing, you'd better be vigilant about whether your structures and processes support consistency of assignments. Once Primary Nurses get to experience the empowerment, autonomy, and depth of connection with patients and families, as well as the ability to do more to improve the patient experience than they ever dreamed possible, you'll meet with significant resistance if you do anything to threaten the continuity of those relationships. For some nurses working in departments where Primary Nursing is done well, the thought of moving to a department or facility that doesn't practice Primary Nursing is completely out of the question.

It is clear from our conversations with Primary Nurses all over the world that nurses and patients benefit equally from this care delivery system. While the benefits to patients and families are covered thoroughly elsewhere in this book, some of the benefits to nurses were beautifully articulated in our interviews with Primary Nurses, and a small sampling is shared here:

Dena Uscio, bba, rn, ocn

The people who were initially such a hard sell on my unit are now some of the biggest supporters of Primary Nursing. I've seen nurses go far above and beyond for their patients. There's personal investment when you're their Primary Nurse. There are definitely boundaries that we don't want to cross as a nurse, but to have personal investment as a nurse—going to see families who have gone to the NICU, or to funerals of patients who have passed, and the family—really, well, we're part of their family.

Kathleen Fowler, bsn, rn

People are switching assignments so they can have their primary patients. Personally, my job satisfaction is better because I get to know these people so well. I get to see the happiness—I get to see the good, the bad. And it really helps me to give them efficient care so that every time my patient comes in I don't have to go over every line of detail, of history, because I know them. Of course I'm going to review it, but it's going to allow me to do my job in a more efficient manner. It decreases my workload and makes it less stressful than if I had to read about every single patient every time.

These Primary Nurses and others understand that practicing in a way that is life-giving for both themselves and their patients requires that they "show up" as fully present participants in their work and their lives, and there are perhaps no words that state more powerfully the act of "showing up" than the words "I am." To say "I am your Primary Nurse" is to commit to being fully alive within your work.

There is still, of course, a place for the "we" in Primary Nursing. *We* design an infrastructure that supports primary relationships for patients and their nurses. *We* cooperate and collaborate to make sure assignments are consistent. *We* learn and grow together. *We* step in, often as a team, to make sure that one Primary Nurse gets the relief he or she needs if the care of one patient and family gets too heavy. All of these situations and more require an exquisite sense of "we" within a department or organization, and each of these expressions of "we" supports the patient and family in their healing.

Finally, though, if the patient and family are to feel held in your care, they must hear you individually step into full responsibility for their care. They must hear you assert your presence in the moment: "I am." And they must hear your commitment to them: "I am your Primary Nurse."

Appendixes

Appendix A

Comparison of the Four Care Delivery Systems Applying the Four Elements

Element	Functional Nursing	Team Nursing	Total Patient Care	Primary Nursing
Nurse–patient relationship and decision making	Decision making occurs over a single shift; decisions are usually made by nurse manager or charge nurse.	Decision making occurs over a single shift; decisions are largely by team leader or nurse manager.	Decision making occurs over a single shift, either by an RN caring for the patient or by a charge nurse.	RN makes decisions for individual patients based on their therapeutic relationship, which is sustained for the length of the stay of the patient on the unit.
Work allocation and/or patient assignments	Nursing assignments are task-based. Nurses are assigned to tasks, rather than to patients.	Nursing assignments are based on level of complexity and commensurate level of expertise; focus is on tasks to be accomplished; assignments change based on patient acuity and work complexity.	Nursing assignments are largely patient-based, with the RN providing activities of care. Nursing assignments may vary by shift based on geography and patient acuity, without supporting continuity of care.	Nursing assignments are patient-based to ensure continuity of care. An RN is assigned to a patient and remains that patient's Primary Nurse for as long as the patient remains on the unit (unless circumstances require that a new Primary Nurse be assigned).

Element	Functional Nursing	Team Nursing	Total Patient Care	Primary Nursing
Communication among health care team members	Communication is hierarchical; task completion is documented and communicated to the charge nurse; the charge nurse pulls information together for all patients and communicates with other members of the heath care team.	Communication is hierarchical; the care provider reports to the team leader; the team leader reports to physicians and/or to other health care team members.	Communication is direct. However, in some Total Patient Care systems, RNs may be required to communicate with the physician and other members of the health care team through a charge nurse.	Communication is direct. Patient information is solicited by the Primary Nurse, who communicates directly and proactively with team members, physicians, and other colleagues. The Primary Nurse is responsible for integrating information and coordinating care.
Management of the unit or environment of care	Managers function as overseers, assuring that tasks are accomplished.	The nurse manager supervises the team leader who is responsible for supervising other staff in the delivery of care.	Managers serve as a resource and promote nurses having a stronger role in care decisions.	Managers promote the nurse–patient relationship and the professional role of the nurse. They influence care by creating a healthy work environment and empowering the staff to remove barriers to care.

Source: From *Relationship-Based Care: A Model for Transforming Practice* (2004), Mary Koloroutis, editor. Used by permission.

Appendix B

Leading Others into Leadership and Ownership: How Nurse Managers Can Support Shared Governance (Without Taking it Over)

GEN GUANCI, MED, RN-BC, CCRN-K

A clear understanding of the role of the nurse manager (or any nurse leader) in a shared governance unit practice council (UPC) is crucial to the individual manager's success as well as the council's. Many times, individuals who are in nurse manager positions are the get-it-done people in an organization. They are able to plan and facilitate or run meetings and get the work done. This type of facilitation, known as basic facilitation, helps a group solve problems by using process skills. This process is a short-term fix in which the group *depends* on the facilitator or nurse manager. Despite the value of this short-term problem solving for some situations, this is exactly what *not* to do as you build a shared governance culture.

The nurse manager's role in building a shared governance culture is as a support or developmental facilitator. This role uses a longer-term strategy in which the team learns how to facilitate its own processes. The nurse manager must help councils function more effectively now and in the future without taking charge of the process. The nurse manager not only helps the council members work on specific issues but encourages them to look at issues from all sides, to see things for themselves, to use their critical thinking, and to come to their own conclusions. In developing a shared governance culture, the nurse manager spends time coaching the members on the process, roles, tools, and techniques before and after the meeting rather than during them. In most situations, the nurse manager does not attend the meetings but may stop in to show visible support and address any questions that may have arisen. The goal of the nurse manager's support, coaching, and mentoring is for the team to develop the skills that enable them to move forward and address the issues of their unit.

The exciting role of the nurse manager is to inspire, model, and advance the council while at the same time helping council members learn to facilitate their own process. Serving as a guide and catalyst, the manager helps people focus their energy while fostering learning, creativity, productivity, and ownership.

Desired Outcomes of the Shared Governance Process

The first step for any group is to determine the desired outcomes. For a shared governance UPC, the desired outcome is acceptance of the responsibility, authority, and accountability (R+A+A) for nursing practice and the outcomes associated with that practice for their nursing unit. These outcomes include patient satisfaction, nurse-sensitive indicator outcomes, and RN satisfaction. Even though the nurse manager may have hopes and dreams for the council, these are not nearly as important as the hopes and dreams the council members have for themselves. My colleagues and I have seen time and time again that nurse managers realize after the fact that unit staff members respond to and adopt what the UPCs come up with much sooner and with less resistance than they would have with the nurse manager's plan for the unit.

Expectations of Nurse Managers in Supporting Their UPCs

- Provide time for UPC members to attend meetings.

- Obtain a schedule of all UPC meetings.

- Review all UPC meeting minutes.

- Support the chair/co-chair in agenda development.

- Empower UPC members.

- Clearly articulate expectations of what the UPC can and cannot make decisions about, as well as the criteria that each decision has to meet and within what time frame.

- Foster a culture of accountability for yourself and the council chair/co-chair and members.

- Meet with the chair/co-chair before meetings to review agenda and any boundaries which the council needs to know about before they begin their work or make decisions.

- Give authority.

- Coach the chair/co-chair to work through any anticipated issues or problems.

- Provide tools to complete unit projects.

- Allow staff to try things that may not work.

- Meet with the chair/co-chair after meetings to debrief, offer feedback and coach for skill development.

- Manage any attempts on the part of the chair/co-chair to defer meeting management to you. This is not your council, not your meeting.

- Get out of the way.

- *Allow* change.

- Celebrate successes.

By supporting your staff as they form and grow their UPC, you will also see the individuals grow personally and professionally as well. What better reward is there for leaders than to watch their staff blossom?

Appendix C

Unit Practice Council Worksheets for Primary Nursing Planning

Instructions

Council members are to engage in dialogue as they answer all the worksheet questions that are relevant to their department. Questions that are not applicable should be skipped. As the answers to questions are determined, the implementation plan for Primary Nursing is being developed. Council members must obtain input from all of their co-workers every step of the way using their communication network.

The majority of the Primary Nursing implementation action plan is created by the UPC without the direct input of the nurse manager. The members of the UPC should independently answer the questions related to the first three elements of the care delivery system: responsibility for the relationship and decision making, work allocation and patient assignments, and communication with the care team. The manager is to be invited into a more direct level of participation when the fourth element of the care delivery system, leadership/management, is discussed.

Element 1: Responsibility for Relationship and Decision Making

One registered nurse accepts responsibility, authority, and accountability for managing the nursing care of specific patients.

Principles

1. One registered nurse (the Primary Nurse) develops a therapeutic relationship and individualized plan of care with the patient and family for their episode of care or service.

2. The patient and family are able to identify their Primary Nurse by name and understand that he or she is responsible for planning and coordinating their care.

3. Registered nurses are accountable for making decisions about the patient's care and for delivering or delegating activities of care and for effectively communicating those decisions to others, assuring smooth handoffs.

4. Other nurses caring for the patient in the absence of the Primary Nurse are responsible for following the plan of care developed by the Primary Nurse or to revise it based on the patient's response and changing needs.

5. Nursing roles are designed to fulfill the scope of practice statements in the state's Nurse Practice Act and to carry out their professional responsibilities.

Questions

What is the nature of the Primary Nurse relationship?

- What kinds of questions will the Primary Nurse use to begin to know the patient as a person?

- What will facilitate the Primary Nurse's ability to be present and attuned to the patient and family?

- Does education on therapeutic relationships need to be provided? If so, who will be responsible for providing education? How will you know when nurses understand this relationship?

- How will what is learned about the patient as a person (and his or her preferences) be communicated to the next caregiver?

What will it mean to be responsible for managing a patient's care for their entire episode of care?

- In what ways will the Primary Nurse demonstrate his or her responsibilities for managing care for his or her primary patients in this department?

- When can other nurses make decisions regarding the patient's plan of care (POC)?

- How will these POC changes be communicated to the Primary Nurse?

Who will serve as Primary Nurses in this department?

- Will all RNs be eligible to be a Primary Nurse? If not, what factors would exclude an RN from participating in this role?

- How will supplemental, float, or PRN staff be used? Under what circumstances?

How will Associate Nurses be identified for each patient?

- How can associate nurses support the relationship between the patient and the Primary Nurse?

- What will the role of associate nurses be?

- When, if ever, will the associate nurse provide the direct patient care when the Primary Nurse is on duty?

- How will the associate nurse role be described to staff, to patients, and to other members of the health care team in order to communicate an appropriate level of expertise and significance?

How will each patient be assigned a Primary Nurse?

- Who is (are) the best person(s) to make this decision?

- What are all the criteria for assigning Primary Nurses (e.g., schedule, patient length of stay, nurse preferences, skill level, frequency of clinic visits, procedures needed)?

- How soon after admission or entry into the care setting should the assignment be made?

- Should there be a maximum number of primary patients that a Primary Nurse has at any one time? What considerations need to be taken into account?

How will the Primary Nurse explain his or her relationship with the patient and family?

- How will the Primary Nurse introduce him- or herself and explain the role and how it is different from other caregivers? Will there be a template or cues as to what to include in the explanation of the Primary Nurse role?

- How will physicians and individuals in other disciplines be informed of the name and responsibilities of the Primary Nurse?

- How will the effectiveness of the communication by the Primary Nurse about their role be measured?

What steps will the Primary Nurse take to complete an individualized assessment and plan of care?

- How will the patient and family be involved in decision making and establishing the goals and plan of care?

- How will the Primary Nurse get input from other caregivers for the plan of care?

- Where is the care plan recorded so that it is available to all caregivers in all disciplines?

- Who will update the plan of care? How will the patient and family be included in the evaluating/updating process?

How will the Primary Nurse communicate the plan of care?

- How will the plan of care be communicated to other members of the team?

- How will the plan be used in report? When transferring a patient to another setting? Between inpatient and outpatient settings?

- Will any components of the plan of care be written on the patient's whiteboard or other visible areas in the care environment?

Once decisions are made and recorded by the Primary Nurse, under what circumstances can others make changes?

- Under what circumstances should others make changes to decisions when the Primary Nurse is not available for input?

- What effect, if any, will this have on the authority of the Primary Nurse?

- What action will be taken if the Primary Nurse leaves no instructions?

Who is currently responsible for discharge planning/care transition, and what is the role of the Primary Nurse in meeting this responsibility?

- Is teaching part of the daily care or clinic visit for the patient?

- How will information be gathered from the patient/family to ensure appropriate discharge planning or transitions to another setting? Who will be responsible for gathering information? How will this information be recorded and shared?

Under what circumstances is it appropriate for the Primary Nurse assignment to be changed?

- What is the process for reassigning a patient to a new Primary Nurse? Who will/can make the decision to reassign a patient to a new Primary Nurse?

- Under what rare circumstances is it appropriate for care to be assigned to another person when the Primary Nurse is on duty? How can this be minimized?

- If a Primary Nurse is on duty and not caring for his or her primary patient, what responsibility does this person have to interact with the patient or family, address discharge/transition needs, or update the plan of care?

Element 2: Work Allocation and Patient Assignments

The registered nurse has full authority for determining the kind and amount of nursing care a patient will receive, as well as who will deliver that care.

Principles

1. Patient assignments are based on the continuity of relationships, the complexity of care required, and the skills and knowledge of the caregiver.

2. Registered nurses have the authority for determining the kind and amount of nursing care a patient will receive, the work that care requires, how much of that work requires the expertise and time of the registered nurse, and how much can be delegated to other caregivers.

Questions

How will assignments be made to support Primary Nursing and continuity of relationships?

- How should the following considerations be prioritized for making shift/clinic assignments: Primary Nurse, prior relationship with the patient or family, skill/knowledge of the nurse/caregiver, patient acuity/safety, workload, room location? (Add other factors as appropriate.)

- What changes could be made to make continuity of assignments the norm?

- How will educational opportunities be provided for the growth and development of newer staff members preparing to be Primary Nurses (e.g. precepting, mentoring)?

- How will it we ensure that staff schedules reflect a healthy balance of a patient-centric focus and self-care considerations?

How will patient assignments be communicated to everyone who needs to know them?

- What new systems will be needed to record and communicate patient assignments and Primary Nurse assignments?

- Are there currently department norms about what work must be done on what shift or day of the week? Do these norms serve the patient or the nurses?

- Will the nurse (Primary or associate nurse) be supported in making decisions in the best interest of the patient and using his or her common sense, rather than making decisions based on previous norms?

- Does one shift or work team criticize another shift or work team for their choices about what is done and what is left undone? If so, how will this be addressed to encourage collaboration rather than competition between the shifts or work teams?

What work needs to be done only by RNs within the context of the Nurse Practice Act, regulatory standards, and hospital policies?

- What does your Nurse Practice Act (NPA) say about the RN role? The LPN role?

- Are all members of the nursing staff familiar with the NPA? How will you educate yourself and others on the scope of practice definitions within your NPA?

- Are there different expectations for RNs, new graduates, and student nurses as:

  » The Primary Nurse?

  » The associate nurse?

- What non-value-added work could be eliminated from nursing?

- What proactive structures and processes could be put in place to ensure that the correct person is taking responsibility for the work?

- For unit clerks/secretaries, what limits to work assignments are imposed by job descriptions? Are they necessary?

Do RNs have full authority to make delegation decisions within external standards such as practice acts and regulatory agencies?

- Are there internal policies that interfere with decisions by the RN regarding delegation?

- How do RNs make thoughtful decisions about when it is in the patient's best interest to do care themselves that is often delegated?

- How do RNs analyze the knowledge and life experience of assistive caregivers to determine whether they are capable of doing a task before delegating it?

- Are assistive personnel utilized to perform all the care they are skilled to do? Could their skills be used more fully?

- Do RNs help teach new knowledge to assistive personnel? What would encourage this practice to take place even more often?

How could Primary Nurses, associate nurses, LPNs, and unlicensed staff be configured in care pairs or partnerships to work consistently with one another and patients?

- How many care pairs or partnerships could be supported on this unit?

- How will the nursing staff be informed about or invited into the partnership concept?

- How can care pairs or partnerships be used to maximize the contributions of assistive personnel?

Do LPNs have an RN assigned to their patients to oversee and manage care?

- If an RN is assigned to a patient for whom an LPN is providing care, what processes/practices will be used to ensure that the RN is managing the patient's care?

- How can care pairs or partnerships be used to maximize the contribution of LPNs?

What scheduling practices need to be maintained or changed in this department to provide for continuity of care?

- Before scheduled days off, how will the Primary Nurse let the patient know who will be caring for him or her?

- Does the department have multiple shift configurations? Can we move to having the same length of shift for all or at least matching schedules of those with 12- and 8-hour shifts to minimize fragmentation?

- Could the number of single shifts worked be reduced?

- How can part-time staff member's work schedules be coordinated to work with a consistent team?

- How is floating handled? How might floating decisions be made to ensure that the patient's best interest is met?

What systems are in place to cover patient care during meals and breaks?

- What are the work area's current systems? Are they working well?

- What is the department culture around meals and other break? Are people supported to take time to eat and rejuvenate? Are staff members criticized when they take this time?

- What may need to be changed?

- If care pairs or partners are used, should they be on break at the same time?

- If care pairs or partners are not used, should there be a buddy system for break/lunch coverage?

Element 3: Communication with the Health Care Team

The registered nurse coordinates communication between the patient and family and members of the interdisciplinary team.

Principles

1. The Primary Nurse proactively seeks information and provides information to others involved in the care of the patient and family.

2. The Primary Nurse coordinates communication between the patient and family and other members of the interdisciplinary team.

3. As the nurse–patient relationship is established, the insight gained into what matters most to specific patients is communicated to other members of the team in order to ensure that care needs and preferences are met.

Questions

What systems will the Primary Nurse use to communicate and coordinate the nursing plan of care with other members of the nursing team and with physicians and clinicians in other disciplines?

- How can the Primary Nurse efficiently gather information or suggestions about the patient from other team members?

- How will the Primary Nurse communicate patient preferences and care decisions to other team members?

- How can the patient and family be kept in the communication loop, receiving timely and consistent information about the plan of care and upcoming activities?

- What structure is or will be in place to ensure that the patient and family are able to contribute information, especially in the absence of the Primary Nurse? How will the structure be communicated to the patient/family?

What processes are in place to ensure communication between patient visits?

- What guidelines exist or need to be developed to ensure that vital information is recorded for follow-up on the next visit?

- How do clinicians in different disciplines communicate during a visit and at subsequent patient encounters?

What communication tools are needed to support continuity of care across settings? How will the electronic medical record be used to support communication?

- How can communication be streamlined to prevent redundancies and fragmentation?

- What method will be used to pass along essential information (e.g., e-messages, one-to-one, written notes)?

- What changes may be needed to enable the Primary Nurse and other key caregivers to communicate regularly about the plan of care?

- How will patients be included in updates/changes/discussions regarding their care?

- Will the whiteboard be a means of communication between the patient/family and the health care team? Will there be other in-room modes of communication?

How effective is shift or team reporting in conveying needed information and involving patients?

- Are there guidelines for reporting? Are they effective?

- How long is reporting? How long should it be?

- Are staff members aware of the advantages of walking rounds and bedside or stretcher-side reporting from the patient's perspective?

- Is the patient and, when appropriate, the family included in reporting? How can this be done most effectively?

- What processes need to be put in place to ensure successful rounds, report, and handoffs that involve the patient?

What specific activities will strengthen collaboration with physicians and clinicians in other disciplines?

- How are communications with the medical staff handled?

- What current practices are effective?

- What will need to change?

- How can RNs and physicians be linked more consistently?

- What changes are needed to allow the primary or associate nurse, the patient, and the physician to meet periodically to discuss the plan of care? What clinicians from other disciplines, if any, should be part of these meetings?

- How can Primary Nurses be involved in physician rounds or visits and interdisciplinary conferences?

Element 4: Leadership/Management

The manager creates an environment that inspires healthy team relationships, professional nursing practice, and the provision of competent and compassionate care.

Principles

1. Managers articulate expectations for an environment in which healthy relationships thrive.

2. The manager promotes professional nursing practice in which registered nurses are autonomous decision makers and creative, empowered problem solvers.

3. The manager leads by inspiring, listening, coaching, and mentoring staff members to promote their professional growth and development.

Questions

Note: The manager should be invited to attend the council meeting in which these questions are discussed.

How will the manager and staff create a shared vision for Primary Nursing in this department?

- How will we create a vision that expresses what the patient will experience in a Primary Nurse relationship?

- What does the council imagine for nurses as they experience this role? What will nurses experience as they take ownership for planning care that is truly personalized?

- How can this vision be used to guide the development of the implementation plan?

- How can this vision be used to help educate all staff about the potential of Primary Nursing?

- How will this vision be described in practical ways?

How can positive caring relationships and collaboration be strengthened?

- What are the standards for how care team members treat each other in this department?

- How will we ensure that everyone follows these standards?

- What education and skill building are needed to build collaboration and effective conflict resolution among all team members?

- How will relationships with colleagues in other departments be optimized?

- What is needed from the manager (skill development opportunities, clearly articulated expectations and follow-through, celebration of achievements, etc.) to assist staff to manage their relationships?

- How will communication with the manager occur to share what is needed?

How can the department manager be most supportive of professional practice?

- How can the manager be most helpful in the implementation of Primary Nursing as the care delivery system?

- How can the manager be most helpful in reinforcing professional practice?

- How can the educator or clinical nurse specialist/leader be most helpful and demonstrate support?

- What is needed from the manager for reinforcement of the Primary Nurse's responsibility for making decisions about the nursing care required for their patients?

How can the voice and needs of staff members be heard and valued?

- How can the manager support the success of his or her UPC?

- How will the manager help UPC members to communicate with 100% of staff?

- What specific support is needed to create a healthy work environment so that caregivers are centered, energized, and inspired to give compassionate care?

- What support does the manager need from administration regarding shared leadership, leading change, and the growth and development of staff members?

What additional education is needed to support therapeutic relationships and Primary Nursing?

- Who can staff members ask for help with this education?

Council members should keep a record of their decisions and gradually summarize these into the department-specific plan for Primary Nursing. When you are finished, return to the UPC chapter to review the sections on education, outcomes and implementation.

Appendix D

Whiteboard Example for Primary Nursing

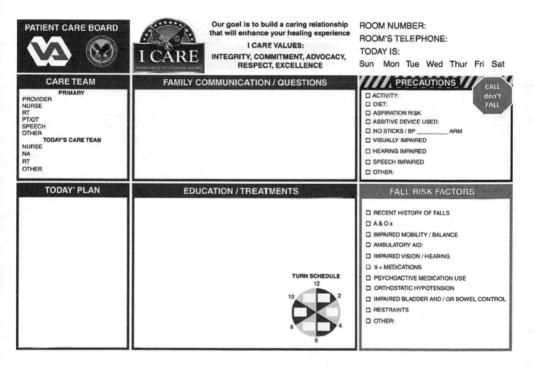

Used with permission. This tool was developed by the Cincinnati VA Medical Center, Unit 6 North UPC. This content is in the public domain and is not under Creative Health Care Management's copyright.

Appendix E

Commitment to My Co-worker© Healthy Team Assessment Survey

Read each of the following statements and rate it on a scale of 1–7 based on how often it is true for you (column 1) and for your team as a whole (column 2):

   1 = Almost never, **2** = Rarely, **3** = Once in a while, **4** = Frequently,
        5 = Quite often, **6**=Usually, **7** = Almost always

Self Team

_____ _____ I believe that it is less important that I "like" my colleagues and more important for us to be committed to the same purpose and goals. (My team believes that it is less important that we "like" one another and more important for us to be committed to the same purpose.)

_____ _____ I accept responsibility for establishing and maintaining healthy interpersonal relationships with my work team members.

_____ _____ I speak directly and promptly with the person involved in a conflict or problem.

_____ _____ I trust my co-workers to do the job they are required and prepared to do.

_____ _____ I address the situation directly and constructively whenever I see a problem in the quality of work.

_____ _____ I respect my colleagues without consideration for titles, education, or job position.

_____ _____ I require my colleagues to treat me with respect.

_____ _____ I address any behavior I perceive as disrespectful or abusive to others or to myself.

_____ _____ I avoid engaging in the "3 Bs": bickering, backbiting, and blaming.

_____ _____ I practice the "3 Cs" in my colleague relationships: caring, committing, and collaborating.

_____ _____ I affirm and recognize my colleagues for quality work.

_____ _____ I avoid complaining about my colleagues; if I have a complaint, I address it with the person.

_____ _____ I avoid gossip.

_____ _____ If I hear someone complaining about another, I will ask that person to speak directly to the other.

_____ _____ I accept others and myself as imperfect—a work (masterpiece) in progress!

_____ _____ Total Score

_____ _____ Average Score (Total/15)

Complete the following statements.

1. I believe our team excels at:

_____

_____

_____

_____

2. I would like to see us build on our already excellent ability to:

_____

_____

_____

_____

I think we can accomplish this by:

_____

_____

_____

_____

3. I think we need strengthening in the area(s) of:

_____

_____

_____

_____

I think we can accomplish this by:

_____

_____

_____

_____

(Koloroutis, 2002)

Appendix F

Example of a Case Presentation

Patient Social Situation

- Patient: 46-year-old male veteran, divorced after 19 years of marriage.

- Two children, a son 18 and living with patient, daughter 11 with shared custody.

- Recently lost temporary job after MVA, losing transportation.

- Poor relationship with siblings; good relationship with parents.

- Family unaware of patient's drug habit; patient wants to keep this confidential.

- No support at home.

Medical History

- Past history: HTN, anxiety, depression, bipolar disorder, insomnia, chronic pain, heavy smoker, current addiction to opioids, including IV drug use.

- Motor vehicle accident prior to admission, treated for trauma and fractures at trauma center, transferred to VA for continued recovery, chest tubes in place.

Problems Identified by Primary Nurse

- Chronic back pain

- Lack of social support

- Decreased activity r/t chest tubes

- Financial concerns r/t no job

- Childcare concerns

- Addiction to IV drugs

Nursing Interventions and Impact

Social Support

- Involved social work and mental health program for substance abuse (this continued after discharge).

- Encouraged communication with family.

- Outcome: Family provided help as requested.

Activity

- Increased mobility by adjusting equipment and rearranging room.

- Outcome: Enabled patient to be out of bed more and patient became independent with most ADLs.

Financial Concerns

- Encouraged patient to seek help from trusted family member.

- Continued support from social services.

- Outcome: Patient's father to assist paying bills while patient is hospitalized; nurse spoke with landlord to verify hospitalization.

Childcare Issues

- Encouraged patient to collaborate with ex-wife in care for younger daughter.

- Outcome: Wife caring for daughter, patient's father checked in on older child.

Pain Management & Substance Abuse Treatment

- Primary Nurse reinforced and encouraged treatment plan from substance experts.

- Close collaboration with physician on effective pain management.

- Outcome: Pain scores improved, following treatment for substance recovery.

Final Reflections and Conclusions

- A key to success was learning what was most important to this patient and planning care around those things. Trust developed with the Primary Nurse enabled honesty about complex social issues.

- Periodic reassessment of problems helped identify new issues and allowed ongoing evaluation of patient's satisfaction with nursing interventions.

- Extensive interdisciplinary communication was effective, including relaying plans among different physician specialists to allow coordination.

- Communication of the nursing plan of care via the whiteboard, care plan, and shift report was effective.

Special thanks to coaches for Primary Nursing implementation: Rebecca Beckman, MS, RN, Quality Improvement Coordinator, and Relationship-Based Care Coordinator, Carol Perry, MSN, RN.

Appendix G

Worksheets to Guide the Manager's Role in Primary Nursing

Principle 1

The manager actively supports shared governance and the success of their unit practice council in implementing Primary Nursing.

Questions

How will I enable meetings of the UPC, balancing the needs of patients and the council?

- If another person does the staff schedule, how will I assist the scheduler to ensure that UPC members are able to attend meetings and patient care is covered?

- What resources will I offer to help with meeting space off the unit?

- How will I support good meeting attendance and replacement of members when needed?

- What message will I convey to staff not on the committee? How will I assist if UPC members meet resistance from colleagues about taking time for meetings?

- Will meeting time be paid time?

- Will I approve overtime if needed?

- Will I support meetings off site?

How will I find out what the council needs from me to be successful?
- Is it helpful for me to attend part or all of any UPC meetings?

- How will I ensure that UPCs are informed of all nursing or regulatory standards/policies that need to be incorporated or considered when developing their plan?

- Will UPC members need time at staff meetings to share updates or education?

- How will I reinforce UPC decisions?

- How will I help remove barriers for acceptance of the UPC plans?

How will I follow up on issues or barriers identified by the UPC that are beyond their scope and get them solved?
- How will I ensure staff's ongoing involvement as I'm doing this?

Principle 2

The manager articulates expectations for Primary Nursing based on the plan developed by the UPC. Managers oversee full implementation, taking action to measure, celebrate, and coach staff as needed.

Questions

What are all of my opportunities to communicate, in words and actions, my expectations that Primary Nursing will be fully embraced for all patients?
- In meetings, in writing, during rounds?

- What questions might I ask staff to communicate my expectations and recognize their good work?

- What questions will I ask patients/family to determine whether they are benefiting from a primary relationship?

In what ways can I reinforce the spread of Primary Nursing and learn about the success of nurses in carrying out this new role?

- How will I celebrate successes?

- Will job descriptions articulate expectations for the roles of the Primary and associate nurses?

- How will performance discussions and evaluations capture an individual's success or opportunities:

  » As a Primary Nurse?

  » As an associate nurse?

  » In managing interpersonal relationships?

  » In developing therapeutic relationships?

How can I help and encourage those who are slow to adopt this role?

- What, if any, time frame will be required for all individuals to accept and participate in the UPC action plans?

- What will I expect of UPC members in relationship to colleague accountability?

- At what point do I need to become involved to coach and counsel staff?

Principle 3

The manager promotes professional practice and reinforces the responsibilities of Primary Nurses for:

- Establishing a therapeutic relationship and personalized patient care.

- Developing a plan of care in partnership with the patient.

- Collaborating with people in other professional disciplines.

Questions

How can I assess each individual nurse's success in developing a therapeutic and trusting relationship with patients and families?

- How will I assess whether Primary Nurses have honored the unique needs and preferences of patients and families in planning their care?

How can I observe and reinforce transdisciplinary and interdepartmental communication and collaboration?

Principle 4

The manager establishes clear expectations for a healthy work environment, which includes teamwork, mutual respect, and open, honest communication.

Questions

Has the UPC translated the organization's values and beliefs about interpersonal relationships into specific behavioral expectations?

- Do we have existing standards of behavior that can be used?

- How will the Commitment to my Co-worker© cards be adopted to accomplish this?

How can I convey my expectations that staff will be responsible for managing their interpersonal relationships consistent with our articulated values and beliefs?

In what ways will I reinforce this expectation during:

- Job interviews?

- Unit orientation?

- Staff meetings?

- Manager rounds, patients and staff?

- Performance reviews?

- Other times?

What process will I use to assess and recognize those who are following our behavioral expectations?

- What expectations do I have of the UPC and other staff members to address one another when individuals do not follow the defined behavior expectations?

What process will I use when individuals have a pattern of consistently not following our agreed-upon behaviors?

Principle 5

The manager measures the effectiveness of Primary Nursing on patient safety, the patient experience, and the quality of care. Outcomes are used as a source of reinforcement and inspiration.

Questions

What measures are most important in assessing whether each patient or family experiences the impact of the Primary Nurse relationship?

How will I participate in collecting these outcomes?

- During patient rounds?

- During conversations with staff or staff rounds?

- As I review documentation?

- Other ways?

How will I use outcome data to inspire staff and others?

What will I do if outcomes do not show improvements? How will I assist/ coach UPC members as necessary to address strategies for improved success?

Principle 6

The manager provides and supports learning opportunities to deepen knowledge of Primary Nursing. Staff members are encouraged to continuously improve their practice and reflect on successes and failures as opportunities to learn.

Questions

In what ways will I support and help educate the entire team in practicing Primary Nursing?

- How will I identify and address educational needs identified by others, such as skills in communication, delegation, therapeutic relationship, etc.?

In what ways can we deepen our insights about the primary relationship and model reflective practice?

- In what ways can we use case conferences?

- How will we share our successes with other departments/clinics in the organization and serve as mentors?

NOTES

Appendix H

Sample Primary Nursing Discharge Survey

The following questions are asked of the patient or key family member.
Share the name of your Primary Nurse, if you can.

Name: _____

Yes _____ (named or described), No _____ (not sure)

- How caring and helpful was the relationship with your Primary Nurse on a scale of 1 to 5, with 1 being not caring and helpful and 5 being extremely caring and helpful?

    1   2   3   4   5   (circle a number)

- Were you introduced to your Primary Nurse within 24 hours of your arrival? Yes _____ No _____

- When you arrived, were you asked what was most important to you and your family? Yes _____ No _____

- Did your Primary Nurse, physician, and other care team members meet jointly with you about your care every day? Yes _____ No _____

- Would you like to share something about your experience here that you especially appreciated?

_____

_____

_____

_____

Thank you for your time and consideration!

References

Alpert, H. B., Goldman, L. D., Kilroy, C. M., & Pike, A. W. (1992). Toward an understanding of collaboration. *Nursing Clinics of North America, 27*(1), 47–59.

American Nurses Credentialing Center (ANCC). (2008). Magnet Recognition Program®. Silver Springs, MD: ANCC Publishing.

Berwick, D. (2009). At the International Forum on Quality and Safety in Health Care, Berlin, Germany, published in *BJM Quality and Safety: The International Journal of Healthcare Improvement*, March. http://qualitysafety.bmj.com/content/18/4/e1.full

Bond, S., Bond, J., Fowler, P., & Fall, M. (1991). Evaluating primary nursing. Part 3. *Nursing Standard, 38*(5), 36–39.

Clemence, M. (1966). Existentialism: A philosophy of commitment. *American Journal of Nursing, 66*(3), 500–505.

Manthey, M. (2002). *Staffing: Changing the way we think.* Minneapolis, MN: Creative Health Care Management.

Edmundson, A. (2012). *Teaming: How organizations learn, innovate, and compete in the knowledge economy.* San Francisco: John Wiley & Sons, Inc.

Eisler, R., & Potter, T. (2014). *Transforming interprofessional partnerships: A new framework for nursing and partnership-based health care.* Indianapolis, IN: Sigma Theta Tau International.

Felgen, J. (2007). *I₂E₂: Leading lasting change.* Minneapolis, MN: Creative Health Care Management.

Forstrom, S., & Weydt, A., Eds. (2008). *Work complexity assessment facilitator's manual.* Minneapolis, MN: Creative Health Care Management.

Gardner, K. (1991). A summary of findings of a five-year comparison study of primary and team nursing. *Nursing Research, 40*(2), 113–117.

Gardner, K. G., & Tilbury, M. (1991). A longitudinal cost analysis of primary and team nursing. *Nursing Economics, 9*(2), 97–104.

Koloroutis, M. (2002). *Re-Igniting the spirit of caring journal.* Minneapolis, MN: Creative Health Care Management.

Koloroutis, M., Ed. (2004). *Relationship-Based Care: A model for transforming practice.* Minneapolis, MN: Creative Health Care Management.

Koloroutis, M., & Trout, M. (2012). *See me as a person: Creating therapeutic relationships with patients and their families.* Minneapolis, MN: Creative Health Care Management.

Manthey, M., Ciske, K., Robertson, P., & Harris, I. (1970). Primary Nursing: A return to the concept of "my nurse" and "my patient." *Nursing Forum, 9*(1), 65–84.

Manthey, M. (1989). *Partners-in-practice: A logical extension.* Minneapolis, MN: Creative Health Care Management.

National Council of State Boards of Nursing. (2005). *The five rights of delegation.* Retrieved from https://www.ncsbn.org/Delegation_joint_statement_NCSBN-ANA.pdf

Persky, G., Felgen, J., & Nelson, J. (2012). Measuring caring in Primary Nursing. In J. Nelson & J. Watson (Eds.), *Measuring caring: International research on caritas as healing.* New York: Springer Publishing Company.

Rathert, C., & May, D. R. (2007). Health care work environments, employee satisfaction, and patient safety: Care provider perspectives. *Health Care Management Review, 32*(1), 2–11.

Sellick, K. J., Russell, S., & Beckmann, J. L. (2003). Primary Nursing: An evaluation of its effects on patient perception of care and staff satisfaction. *International Journal of Nursing Studies, 40*(5), 545–551.

Wessel, S. (2012). Impact of unit practice councils on culture and outcomes. *Creative Nursing, 18*(4), 187–192.

Wessel, S., Felgen, J., Person, C., & Kinnaird, L. (2008). *Relationship-Based Care implementation guide.* Minneapolis, MN: Creative Health Care Management.

Zolnierek, C. D. (2014). An integrative review of knowing the patient. *Journal of Nursing Scholarship, 46,* 3–10.

Index

The abbreviation "PN" stands for the term Primary Nursing.

Components of a
Relationship-Based Care Delivery System

The central focus of Relationship–Based Care is the Patient and Family.
All care practices and priorities are organized around
the needs and priorities of patients and families.
Care is experienced when one human being connects with another.

Leaders know the vision, act with purpose, remove barriers, and consistently hold patients, families and staff as their highest priority.

Teamwork requires a group of diverse members from all disciplines and departments to define and embrace a shared purpose and to work together to fulfill that purpose.

Achieving quality outcomes requires planning, precision and perseverance. It begins with defining specific, attainable and measurable outcomes and uses outcome data to continuously enhance performance.

Professional practice integrates compassionate care with clinical knowledge and expertise. Professional nurses work collaboratively with all caregivers, disciplines and departments in the interest of patient care.

Relationship–Based Care
Leadership
Teamwork
Outcomes
Patient & Family
Resources
Professional Practice
Care Delivery
Caring and Healing Environment

A resource driven practice is one which maximizes all available resources, staff, time, equipment, systems and budget.

The patient care delivery system is the infrastructure for organizing and providing care to patients and families. The system determines the way in which the activities of care are accomplished and is built upon the concepts and values of professional nursing practice.

In a caring and healing environment patients, families and colleagues experience care that is attentive to body, mind, and spirit. Caring theory and science informs intentional actions that support self-care, therapeutic relationships with patients, families and healthy peer relationships. Operational practices and physical settings reinforce this commitment to a caring culture.

Consulting Services from Creative Health Care Management:
A Critical Step in a Successful Relationship-Based Care Implementation

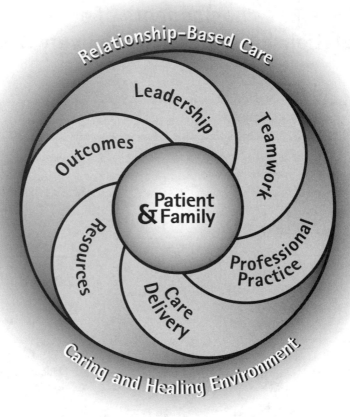

Relationship-Based Care

Leadership

Teamwork

Outcomes

Patient & Family

Resources

Professional Practice

Care Delivery

Caring and Healing Environment

Care Delivery Design for Relationship-Based Care

The core of Relationship-Based Care is implementing a care delivery system that supports:

- Knowing the patient as a person

- Great collaboration among clinicians

- Smooth transitions among caregivers

The care delivery system within RBC is one in which the patient experiences the close attention and care coordination of a "primary caregiver" within each discipline. Based on the time-tested principles of Primary Nursing, this evidence-based care delivery system is effective for inpatient care, outpatient settings, and ambulatory clinics.

Creative Health Care Management has been partnering with organizations to redesign care delivery for over 35 years based on a commitment to strong continuity of care which happens with the greatest consistency when a primary caregiver accepts responsibility for providing personalized, patient-driven care.

Care Delivery Design with Primary Caregivers

Based on the classic work by Marie Manthey on Primary Nursing, and expanded to include caregivers in all professional disciplines, the system of Primary Caregivers enables patients to know who is responsible for coordinating their care within each discipline. One caregiver in each setting or service is designated as Primary Nurse, Primary Therapist, Primary Social Worker, and so on. The implementation of this care delivery system is designed by front line staff and is adapted for each unique care setting. Implementation of Primary Caregivers is directly responsible for important outcomes, including:

- Improved patient experience

- Emotional safety

- Earlier identification of changes in patient's condition

- Reduced workload for clinicians as they care for the same patients

- Better communication among disciplines and with physicians

An essential part of achieving strong quality and a great patient experience is a care delivery system that facilitates exemplary care.

For consultation in Relationship-Based Care and Primary Nursing, go right to the source.

Creative Health Care Management was founded in 1978 by Marie Manthey, one of the originators of Primary Nursing. Since that time, we've helped clients around the world to transform their cultures through the implementation of Primary Nursing and Relationship-Based Care.

Creative Health Care Management empowers, engages, and inspires health care organizations across the world to transform their cultures into those that provide an unmatched experience for their patients and families and colleagues in all disciplines.

We use relationship-based consultation services, innovative education programs, the latest experiential learning methodologies, and some of the most celebrated products in the industry to engage leaders throughout the organization, ultimately empowering those closest to the work in executing their organization's mission and achieving results.

Creative Health Care Management is a women-owned business located in Minneapolis, Minnesota.

Visit **www.chcm.com** for information about how Creative Health Care Management can help you bring your mission to life.

ORDER FORM

1. Order Online at: shop.chcm.com
2. Call toll-free 800.728.7766 x4 and use your Visa, Mastercard, Discover, or American Express or a company purchase order
3. Fax your order to: 952.854.1866
4. Mail your order with pre-payment or company purchase order to:

    Creative Health Care Management
    5610 Rowland Road, Suite 100
    Minneapolis, MN 55343-8905
    Attn: Resources Department

CREATIVE

HEALTH CARE

MANAGEMENT

Product	Price	Quantity	Subtotal	TOTAL
B670 - Primary Nursing: Person Centered Care Delivery System Design	$34.95			
B510 - Relationship-Based Care: A Model for Transforming Practice	$34.95			
B650 - See Me As a Person: Creating Therapeutic Relationships ...	$39.95			
B600 - Relationship-Based Care Field Guide	$99.00			
B560 - I₂E₂: Leading Lasting Change	$24.95			
M501 - Commitment to My Co-worker Cards (pack of 25)	$15.00			
Shipping Costs: Please call 800.728.7766 x4 for a shipping estimate.				
Order TOTAL				

Need more than one copy? We have quantity discounts available.

Quantity Discounts (Books Only)		
10–49 = 10% off	**50–99** = 20% off	**100 or more** = 30% off

Payment Methods: ☐ **Credit Card**   ☐ **Check**   ☐ **Purchase Order PO#** _____

Credit Card	Number	Expiration	AVS# (3 digit)
Visa / Mastercard / Discover / AMEX	– – –	/	
Cardholder address (if different from below):	**Signature:**		

Customer Information	
Name:	
Title:	
Company:	
Address:	
City, State, Zip:	
Daytime Phone:	
Email:	

Satisfaction guarantee: If you are not satisfied with your purchase, simply return the products within 30 days for a full refund.
For a free catalog of all our products, visit shop.chcm.com or call 800.728.7766 x4.